Management in Physiotherapy

EDITED BY
ROBERT J JONES
District Physiotherapy Manager
Eastbourne Health Authority

RADCLIFFE MEDICAL PRESS
OXFORD

1784242 5

© 1991 Radcliffe Medical Press Ltd
15 Kings Meadow, Ferry Hinksey Road, Oxford OX2 0DP

British Library Cataloguing in Publication Data

The management of physiotherapy.
  1. Great Britain. National health services. Physiotherapy
    services. Organization.
  I. Jones, Robert J.
362.178
ISBN 1-870905-81-4

Typeset by Advance Typesetting Ltd, Oxfordshire
Printed in Great Britain by
Billing & Sons Ltd, Worcester

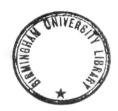

DEDICATION

TO ADAM AND ALISTAIR

Contents

List of Tables

List of Figures

List of Abbreviations

ACAS	Advisory Conciliation and Arbitration Services
AHA	Area Health Authority
BMA	British Medical Association
CMMS	Case-mix Management Systems
.CPSM	Council for the Professions Supplementary to Medicine
CSP	Chartered Society of Physiotherapy
CV	Curriculum Vitae
DA	District Administrator
DCP	District Community Physician
DGH	District General Hospital
DGM	District General Manager
DoH	Department of Health
DHA	District Health Authority
DHSS	Department of Health and Social Security
DMT	District Management Team
DMU	Directly Managed Unit
DPM	District Physiotherapy Manager
DRG	Diagnosis Related Group
EPCA	Employment Protection (Consolidation) Act
FHSA	Family Health Services Authority
FPO	Federation of Professional Organizations
GP	General Practitioner
GWC	General Whitley Council
HAA	Hospital Activity Analysis
HAV	Home Assessment Visit
HC	Health Circular
HIPE	Hospital In-patient Enquiry
HMSO	Her Majesty's Stationery Office
HN	Health Notice
IPR	Individual Performance Review
IR	Industrial Relations
LORS	Locally Organized Research Scheme
MDS	Minimum Data Set
MoH	Ministry of Health
MLSO	Medical Laboratory Scientific Officer
NAQA	National Association of Quality Assurance
NHS	National Health Service
NHSTA	National Health Service Training Authority
OCR	Optical Character Recognition
PAM	Professions Allied to Medicine
PAS	Patient Administration System
PI	Performance Indicator
PIU	Physiotherapy Input Unit

PRIU	Physiotherapy Resource Input Unit
POMR	Problem Orientated Medical Records
PRB	Pay Review Body
PRP	Performance Related Pay
PT'A'	Professional and Technical 'A'
RCN	Royal College of Nursing
RGM	Regional General Manager
RHA	Regional Health Authority
RMI	Resource Management Initiative
RMT	Regional Management Team
SGT	Self-Governing Trust
TUC	Trades Union Congress
UGM	Unit General Manager
UMT	Unit Management Team
WTE	Whole Time Equivalent

Acknowledgements

I would like to thank very sincerely all of the contributors to this book, for the time and effort they spent writing their chapters and for their generous co-operation throughout its preparation. It has been a privilege and pleasure to work with Sheila Philbrook, Andy Andrews, Marcy Holland, Ann Hunter, Brenda Samuels, Maggie Pauling, Chris Bithell and Phil Gray.

My thanks also go to the many other people who have helped in a wide variety of ways, to Gill Jones, Chris Fincham, Phyllis Hoffman, Roland Milner and Marion Graham, who skilfully and patiently typed the manuscript. Thanks to the Superintendent physiotherapists based at Eastbourne DGH for their valuable advice and practical assistance also the physiotherapy staff and the South East Thames Physiotherapy Information Systems and Resource Management Working Group who developed much of the information systems work. To Gillian Nineham and Andrew Bax of Radcliffe Medical Press, many thanks. Stuart Skyte and many others at the Chartered Society of Physiotherapy Headquarters have been very helpful throughout. Particular thanks also to Joyce Williams for very generously allowing me to use some of her diagrams and material.

I acknowledge and gratefully thank them all.

ROBERT J. JONES
October 1990

Contributors

ANDY P. ANDREWS, *Regional Legal Adviser, South East Thames Regional Health Authority*

CHRISTINE P. BITHELL, *Principal Lecturer, Physiotherapy Division, Institute of Health and Rehabilitation, Polytechnic of East London*

PHILLIP H. GRAY, *Director of Industrial Relations, Chartered Society of Physiotherapy; Staff Side Secretary, PT'A' Whitley Council*

MARCY A. HOLLAND, *Physiotherapy Computer Officer, Eastbourne Health Authority*

ANN E. HUNTER, *District Physiotherapist, Bloomsbury Health Authority*

ROBERT J. JONES, *District Physiotherapy Manager, Eastbourne Health Authority; Member, Eastbourne Hospital Executive Board*

MAGGIE PAULING, *Superintendent Physiotherapist, King's College Hospital, London*

SHEILA A. PHILBROOK, *District Physiotherapist, Barking, Havering and Brentwood Health Authority*

BRENDA M. SAMUELS, *District Physiotherapist, Tower Hamlets Health Authority*

Foreword by D. M. INNOCENTI, *Superintendent Physiotherapist, Guy's Hospital, London.*

Disclaimer

The contents of this book do not necessarily represent Chartered Society of Physiotherapy policy.

Foreword

I am delighted that this book has come to fruition. The changes in the National Health Service have come in waves over the past 20 years and physiotherapists have had to be active in responding to them. Many people have seen these upheavals as opportunities and have transformed them into positive steps towards the improvement of our services to the patients, education of the staff and management of the process.

The purpose in publishing this book is to make available some of the results of these activities. Each chapter is an entity in itself and can be used as an encouragement to those who are actively engaged in managing the services, and as a guide for those about to enter and take on these responsibilities.

The text is not a continuous narrative, but a collection of subjects closely linked into the whole. This book, therefore, will serve as a source of information and guidance, allowing the reader to turn to any chapter according to the subject matter required.

I am grateful to the authors of these chapters, and for the corporate work. They have agreed to give of their precious time to commit the consequences of their experiences to paper as a foundation from which to work for the benefit of our profession, our patients and for those who will be following on.

DIANA M. INNOCENTI MCSP
Guy's Hospital

Preface

There is, today, a wide and steadily increasing range of literature on the theory and practice of physiotherapy. There are also many books available on the theory and practice of management, but so far there has been no specific book for physiotherapy managers. It seemed to me that with so many radical changes occurring in the National Health Service (NHS) at present—and these at such a rapid pace—that now is the right time for a book on physiotherapy management.

This book has been written particularly for physiotherapy managers in all grades throughout the NHS. However, I hope that it will also be of use and interest to physiotherapy clinicians and educators as well as other managers in the NHS, especially those in the professions allied to medicine (PAM).

All of the contributors are widely experienced, whether this be in physiotherapy management, industrial relations, legal matters or computing. Although each chapter stands alone in its own right, there are several major strands which bring the different aspects together into an integrated whole.

The job content, duties and responsibilities of the physiotherapy manager form the main focus of the book, much of which stems from the development of physiotherapy as an independent profession, as does clinical autonomy which is strongly linked, and dependent upon, managerial autonomy. Managerial autonomy is the management of physiotherapy by physiotherapists. Other important strands are quality assurance, resource management and information systems, development of research and student clinical education. There are legal and ethical responsibilities and considerations in all 'true' professions; staff management and personnel duties together with sound industrial relations practice, are also of paramount importance. All of these issues are discussed and set in the context of the 'new' NHS and the development of physiotherapy as an independent profession within it.

There is no 'best, right or only one' way of management. The joint aim of myself and all of the contributors has been to point out various approaches which we hope will enhance understanding and help managers to manage their service sensitively, effectively and efficiently, and by so doing, provide the best quality service possible to our patients.

ROBERT J. JONES
October 1990

1 Physiotherapy Management— An Introduction

R.J. Jones

What is a manager?

The question, 'What is a manager?', is difficult to answer with a single definition because there is as wide a variety of management jobs in the economy as there are definitions in the extensive academic literature. However, some of these definitions point the way to an understanding of the job content, duties and responsibilities of the physiotherapy manager.

Mintzberg's 10 roles for the manager are cited in *Understanding Organizations* (Handy 1986).[1] These are inter-personal roles which are figurehead, leader and liaison; informational roles, i.e. monitor, disseminator and spokesman; and finally decisional roles which are entrepreneur, disturbance handler, resource allocator and negotiator. Handy himself uses more colloquial descriptions of the three sets of roles which are leading, administrating and fixing. All of these are central to the management of physiotherapy services in the National Health Service (NHS). Barnard, in his classic treatise entitled *The Functions of the Executive* (Barnard 1938),[2] sets out the functions of the executive—by which he meant all kinds of managers—as being the maintenance of organizational communication, the securing of essential services from individuals in the organization, and the formulation and definition of purpose, i.e. planning. Again, these three functions are essential components in the management of physiotherapy services in integrating the whole and in finding the best balance between conflicting forces and events. Planning and control are seen by Armstrong (1986)[3] to be the two key managerial activities. He recognizes the importance of the part played by management techniques in managerial skills, procedures and activities. Two 'popular' answers to the question, 'What is a manager?' are mentioned in the *Practice of Management* (Drucker 1968).[4] One is that 'management is the people at the top—the term "management" being little more than a euphemism for "the boss"'. The other one defines a manager as 'someone who directs the work of others and who, as the slogan puts it, "does his work by getting other people to do theirs"'. All of these definitions and answers shed some light, but they are inadequate because they do not wholly explain what management is or what managers do. These two questions can only be answered by '. . . analysing management's function. For management is an organ; and organs can be described and defined only through their function' (Drucker 1968).[5]

The approach of describing the function of the Physiotherapy Manager and analysing the job content, duties and responsibilities is the keystone of this book. This is set in the context of physiotherapy as an autonomous profession—the third largest direct patient care profession in the NHS—linking and working with the other health care providers and services, and against a background of radical and rapid change throughout the whole organization.

The job content, duties and responsibilities of the Physiotherapy Manager

During 1987, a postal questionnaire survey of Senior Physiotherapy Managers throughout England and Wales was carried out (Jones 1989).[6] One objective of this survey was to analyse the content of Senior Physiotherapy Manager posts. One questionnaire was posted to the most senior Physiotherapy Manager in each district. See Table 1.1. below. Of the 200 questionnaires posted, 180 (90%) were completed and returned and of these 180, 160 post-holders (88.9%) held the title District Physiotherapist.

Table 1.1.   Response rate to postal questionnaire (England and Wales)

No. of questionnaires posted	200	(100%)
No. of questionnaires completed and returned	180	(90%)
No. of questionnaires returned by District Physiotherapists	160	(80%)
No. of questionnaires returned by non-district post-holders where there was no District Physiotherapist	20	(10%)
Non-responses	20	(10%)

This group of Physiotherapy Managers was asked to indicate the managerial duties and responsibilities which they undertook, and the results for District Physiotherapists are tabulated opposite.

Table 1.2 shows that Physiotherapy Managers have wide-ranging managerial duties and responsibilities, and that a high percentage carry out a substantial personnel management workload. Those management responsibilities with a high level of clinical implication are clearly very substantially undertaken by physiotherapy heads of service; for example the organization of staff rotations through various clinical specialties, Individual Performance Review (IPR), organization of staff post-registration education and training, monitoring services and the management of research projects.

Between April 1987 and March 1988, 17 District Physiotherapy appointments in 11 Regional Health Authorities (RHA) of England and Wales were advertised nationally and the job descriptions were obtained for analysis

Table 1.2. Managerial duties and responsibilities undertaken by District Physiotherapist post-holders

Managerial responsibilities and duties	Percentage of District Physiotherapists undertaking this work
Physiotherapy budget management	86.3
Management of physiotherapy clinical student placements	66.3
Organization of post-registration physiotherapy education	98.8
Hold staff training budget	31.9
Organization of research projects	67.5
Recruitment advertising	87.5
Recruitment interviewing	98.1
Writing job and role descriptions	97.5
Appointment/termination papers	69.4
IPR (staff development/Individual Performance Review appraisal)	95.6
Grievance/disciplinary procedures	91.3
Statistical returns	94.4
Time sheets	84.4
Sick leave returns	89.4
Annual leave returns	91.3
Staff rotations	91.9
Ordering and deployment of equipment	92.5
Ordering uniforms	77.5
Ordering stores	84.4
Physiotherapy development proposals (planning)	98.8
Monitoring services	100.0
Patients audit	68.8
Introducing Körner and information systems	89.4
Management budgeting	56.3
Unit Superintendent responsibility as well as District role	69.4

(Jones 1989).[7] As responses to the main questionnaire were obtained from heads of District physiotherapy services, this small supplementary study was undertaken in order to ascertain District Health Authority (DHA) requirements for their senior physiotherapy management posts.

The job descriptions were broken down and sorted into key function areas and the figures were collated to show how many Authorities required duties and responsibilities to be undertaken in each of these work areas. The results of this analysis are shown in Table 1.3 overleaf.

Table 1.3.   District Health Authority requirements for job content—Senior
Physiotherapy Manager posts (percentage in parentheses)

Content of post	Number of DHAs requiring this
Manage District Service	17 (100.0)
Manage a Clinical Unit as well as District Service	15 (88.2)
Undertake some clinical work	13 (76.4)
Professional leadership	15 (88.2)
Professional standards and clinical practice	16 (94.1)
Manage budget and other resources	15 (88.2)
Personnel	
Recruitment procedures	16 (94.1)
Counselling	15 (88.2)
IPR (appraisal, career development)	17 (100.0)
Disciplinary and grievance	15 (88.2)
Health/safety	13 (76.4)
Training needs	17 (100.0)
Encourage research	14 (82.3)
Liaising with:	
Training schools	10 (58.8)
Organizations outside NHS	13 (76.4)
Heads of other services, medical staff, managers	17 (100.0)
Input to DHA	17 (100.0)
Planning teams and committee work	8 (47.0)
Manpower and finance planning	17 (100.0)
Physiotherapy policy/strategy	12 (70.5)
Service review and monitoring—standards	17 (100.0)
Quality assurance	10 (58.8)
Staff deployment	15 (88.2)
Information systems, statistics, Körner, etc.	13 (76.4)
Implementation of HA policies	9 (52.9)
Implementation of national/DHSS policies	8 (47.0)
Total HAs included	17 = 100.0

A requirement in all cases was management of the District physiotherapy
service. Other duties which all DHAs mentioned were IPR, training
strategies, liaising with other disciplines, service review and monitoring
and planning. Personnel duties ranked highly, as did clinical work and
responsibility for managing a clinical area (as well as the District service).
Professional leadership, together with professional standards and clinical
practice, were also important in the view of Health Authorities. Most

post-holders were required to be responsible for managing the physiotherapy budget and other resources.

These data strongly support the information provided by the Senior Physiotherapy Managers in the questionnaire survey (Table 1.2) and confirm that they undertake a full managerial workload as clinical heads of this clinical service.

The relationship between the findings of the questionnaire and the analysis of job descriptions is shown in Table 1.4.

Table 1.4. A comparison of findings from the questionnaire survey and job description

Item of job content and responsibility	Senior Physiotherapy Managers' questionnaires	Analysis of DHA job descriptions
Manage budget	86.3	88.2
Planning	98.8	100.0
Monitor service	100.0	100.0
Recruitment procedures	92.8	94.1
IPR	95.6	100.0
Deployment of staff	70.0	88.2
Training needs/post-registration education	98.8	100.0

The information in Tables 1.2, 1.3 and 1.4 shows the diversity of duties and responsibilities in senior physiotherapy management, and this is reflected to some extent in Superintendent and senior posts at all levels.

Clearly, management decisions and actions in all of these areas relate to clinical matters and are therefore directly concerned with patient care.

In view of the NHS reforms resulting from the Prime Minister's National Health Service Review and Government White Paper *Working for Patients* (*see* Chapter 5), there will be a wide range of new and demanding duties for Physiotherapy Managers, as well as a significant expansion of existing ones. A new and complex area of work will be participation in the contracting process, and developing and agreeing contract specifications for the provision of physiotherapy services. Some of the other responsibilities will be more detailed work on quality assurance (*see* Chapter 9), including the development of outcome measures, audit and standards. It will be necessary to become more involved in resource management initiative projects, including the development of information systems, clinical case mix, staffing and grade mix, financial forecasts, costing and service pricing (*see* Chapter 7). It is also likely that Physiotherapy Managers will be required to work on projects in business planning, income generation and marketing.

In some Districts, they may be asked to act on behalf of the DHA (Commissioning Authority), rather than the service provider, in the production of purchasing specifications which describe the services authorities wish to buy for their resident populations.

Physiotherapists are employed in a wide range of clinical areas within the NHS, including the developing specialties (for physiotherapy) of special needs/learning difficulties, mental illness and community care. Modern physiotherapy has a wide scope and spectrum of practice which crosses all unit boundaries.

The Senior Physiotherapy Manager participants in the questionnaire survey (Jones 1989)[8] were asked how many whole time equivalent (WTE) staff were employed in each of the main care group areas in their districts. All of the respondents answering this section stated that physiotherapists were employed in each of the care groups. Table 1.5 shows the average number of WTE staff in each care group in the 160 districts of England and Wales which responded.

Table 1.5. Average WTE physiotherapy staffing in care groups

Care group	Average number of WTE physiotherapists in each care group
Acute	24.02
Mental illness	2.7
Special needs/learning difficulties	2.7
Community domiciliary	4.18
Paediatric and school health	5.4
Elderly care	8.0
Out-patients/gymnasium (including GP open access)	12.1
Obstetrics and gynaecology	2.8
Other (including health promotion/education)	7.1

To achieve the maximum effectiveness of physiotherapy interventions and a co-ordinated service to patients across all unit boundaries, an overview with good communication throughout the service is necessary. Physiotherapy Managers are responsible for ensuring the optimum use of limited manpower and all other resources, they act as catalysts to initiate and develop new fields of service, and widen the service provision, forging stronger links with a wide range of agencies both inside and outside the NHS.

Effectiveness and efficiency

'Value for money' is a frequently repeated phrase in relation to public services, industries and businesses of all types including the NHS and, in common with other services, this requirement is central to the management of physiotherapy. Optimum value for money for patients and tax payers is obtainable only through maximizing effectiveness and efficiency within the service, and it is the management of an effective and efficient service, in all its aspects, that is the core of the Physiotherapy Manager's job.

Effectiveness and efficiency are two quite distinct concepts. Effectiveness relates to the clinical outcomes of service provision, whilst efficiency is concerned with maximizing the outputs from a given set of inputs. In order to measure effectiveness, objectives must first be set in clinical and managerial areas. Goals are set by individual physiotherapists for their individual patients, for example to enable an immobile patient to become mobile again or, in the case of a child with cerebral palsy, to enable independent sitting, to achieve independent feeding, to enable a child to stand from the sitting position and to achieve sufficient manual dexterity for independent dressing. In terms of management, goals are set for the service as a whole or parts such as units or sections. The next step is to devise a method of measuring the degree to which these objectives are met. The level of success in achieving these goals is evaluated on a time scale so as to give a measure of outcome; further goals are then set. The summation of clinical outcomes measured against the expected outcomes is an important clinical and managerial tool. Managerially, this may relate to the possible options concerning the use of physiotherapy staff resources. It might, for example, be judged that the physiotherapy staff time is better spent in taking children's group activities rather than treating individuals on a one-to-one basis. Managerially, at Unit or District level, the Senior Physiotherapy Manager agrees a series of aims and objectives for the Unit or District service. These aims and objectives are agreed in relation to particular care groups and specific clinical areas, as well as for administrative and managerial tasks, and relate to overall Unit or DHA objectives (Figure 1.1). Figure 1.1 (Williams 1986)[9] represents the way in which performance at the level of individual interventions adds up to overall performance at unit or district level.

The effectiveness of the section, Unit or District physiotherapy service is calculated by the summation of the effectiveness of all its parts. An important task for the Physiotherapy Manager is to work towards the development of the relevant outcome measures which are necessary to achieve the balance of resources needed for the agreed and optimum use of finances.

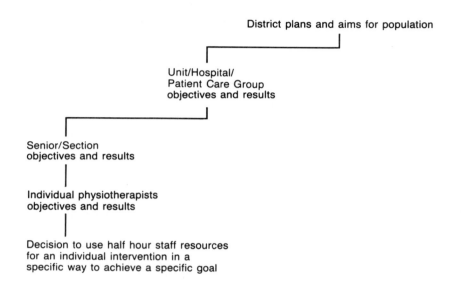

District plans and aims for population

Unit/Hospital/
Patient Care Group
objectives and results

Senior/Section
objectives and results

Individual physiotherapists
objectives and results

Decision to use half hour staff resources
for an individual intervention in a
specific way to achieve a specific goal

Figure 1.1.   Hierarchy of measures of effectiveness

The concept of effectiveness is inextricably linked with that of efficiency. Whereas effectiveness is concerned with the outcomes resulting from physiotherapy intervention, efficiency is 'measured by the ratio of inputs in the medical service provided. The greater the outputs from a given set of inputs, the greater is the efficiency' (Brooks 1986).[10]

A further useful definition is to consider 'effectiveness as referring to achieving maximum professional and clinical outcomes and efficiency as doing so at least cost' (Williams 1986).[11] This definition encompasses the concept of a ratio of inputs to outputs, i.e. the idea of maximizing outputs from the allocated resources.

Physiotherapy resource inputs include:

- *Revenue spending*: workforce input, travel costs, consumables, printing, energy and others.
- *Capital*: buildings, facilities and equipment.

One of the tasks of the Physiotherapy Manager is to ensure, as far as possible, the efficient use of resources in order to achieve optimum outcomes, i.e. service effectiveness. There are many factors involved in achieving efficiency in physiotherapy provision; listed overleaf is a summary of the most important ones.

Staff time spent treating patients	Treatment priority of most urgent patients
Planning and scheduling the working day	Monitoring patient non-attendance in out-patients
Caseload adjustment	Use of diary appointment systems
Comparison of staff caseloads	Patients advised how to continue at home
Avoidance of unnecessary overtime	Optimum use of space
Prioritizing problems	Time-tabling of busy equipment
Efficient skill use (teaching other carers where appropriate)	Arranging relevant postgraduate staff training
Thorough clinical assessment	Planning travel in the community
Thorough record keeping system	Simple and relevant paperwork systems
Patient discharge at appropriate time	Most effective use of skilled staff
Monitoring changes in referral patterns	Monitoring of staff absence
Accessibility of adequate equipment	Physiotherapy staff use as teaching resource
Optimum skill mix appropriate to task	
Monitoring objectives and outcomes	Monitoring of overtime, 'on-call' and travel costs
Caseload priority (when staff absent)	
Waiting list times (why?)	Analysis of monthly turnover figures (throughput)

(Williams 1986)[12]

Figure 1.2. Factors involved in achieving efficiency

Many of these factors can be measured, giving the Physiotherapy Manager an important management tool. Clearly, one aim of the Physiotherapy Manager must be to ensure service efficiency and effectiveness, and this is an integral part of the managerial process.

Accountability

A further responsibility of the physiotherapy manager is to be accountable for the service provision within the terms laid down by the employing authority and jointly agreed. To be accountable is to be required by a specified person, group or organization to report on and justify (give account for) actions in relation to specified matters. Accountability for and within physiotherapy services, in common with many other departments in the NHS, is multi-factorial.

Firstly, there is the physiotherapist's accountability to his/her patients for high standards of therapeutic practice and behaviour. Patients are frequently not in a position, or may not be inclined, to require that the physiotherapist justifies actions on specified matters relating to practice. Therefore, the

Physiotherapy Manager is the first arbiter in professional matters within the service and is the individual to whom the physiotherapists are accountable, in this the Physiotherapy Manager acts as agent for the employer. There are numerous activities for which the physiotherapist is accountable to the Physiotherapy Manager; for example the collection of statistical information, keeping full and accurate treatment records, and attending relevant ward rounds and case conferences, as well as undertaking the relevant caseload. In turn, the most senior Physiotherapy Manager is accountable to the employer for the provision of an efficient and effective service.

Professional accountability cannot be divorced from the control of the resources deployed in effective patient care. Some Health Authorities have opted for a system of split accountability whereby the manager of physiotherapy services is accountable to one officer managerially and another professionally. However, this option may cause confusion and result in uncertainty on the part of all three officers because professional and managerial decisions are synonymous with one another. Most management decisions in physiotherapy are concerned with clinical matters; for example the delegation of a balanced and manageable caseload for a newly qualified physiotherapist or for a small team of staff working in a particular clinical unit. Clearly, accountability impinges on both professional and managerial areas, and the two are inextricably linked.

An analysis of the job content, duties and responsibilities of the senior Physiotherapy Manager is the key to an understanding of the management process and the work of Physiotherapy Managers in the context of physiotherapy itself and the NHS as a whole. An outline of the major management functions clearly demonstrates the interdependence and integrated relationship of the clinical, professional and managerial aspects of the work. The post-holders are the professional and clinical heads of service with an overall management function and the amalgamation of these three strands is essential to maximizing effectiveness and efficiency in the service. Clearly, therefore, there would be very substantial barriers to the effective and efficient management of the service if it were managed by a person other than a physiotherapist. It is the senior Physiotherapy Manager who is accountable for the most effective and efficient service within agreed or available resources.

2 Professionalization
R.J. Jones

The title 'Health Profession' embraces many of the occupational groups in health care provision; physiotherapy is one such group. The growth of professionalization and occupational development have had an important influence on the way in which physiotherapy services have been managed in the NHS. The process of professionalization is an important reason why physiotherapy services are managed by a physiotherapist in the majority of DHAs. The introduction of general management with the unitization of services under the management of Unit General Managers (UGMs)—who could come from any background in or outside the NHS (*see* Chapter 4)—and the Government White Paper *Working for Patients* (*see* Chapter 5) has opened up a debate about the most effective and efficient way to manage and provide this service.

What is a profession?

Exactly what constitutes a profession is a complex issue. The term may be used in both descriptive and evaluative senses. Friedson (1970)[1] distinguished between the structural element of professional status and that concerned with values and attitudes—professionalism. An exploration of the question of whether physiotherapy is a profession or not indicates aspects of physiotherapy practice which are of importance to the way physiotherapy services are managed and organized.

There is a vast literature on the sociology of the profession, most of it American in origin. One of the early works on the topic was a study which concluded that a profession was a complex of characteristics (Carr-Saunders & Wilson 1933).[2] The acknowledged 'ideal' professions of law and medicine exhibited all or most of these features. The features to which they referred were: (1) a technique acquired by prolonged and intellectual training which enabled them to provide a specialized service and (2) the development of an association which imposed tests of competence and required the observance of certain standards of conduct. This model was conceived in the static terms of the definable characteristics or traits which accepted professions possessed. However, Carr-Saunders & Wilson accepted that other occupational groups may have been in the process of developing some of these characteristics.

Five attributes for a profession were proposed (Greenwood 1975).[3]

1 Systematic theory.
2 Authority.
3 Community sanction.
4 Ethical code.
5 A culture of professional knowledge, behaviour and ethos.

A developmental sequence of professionalization was proposed (Wilensky 1964)[4] in which the first step was to start doing full time the thing that needed doing; setting up a new area of practice recruited from other occupational groups. This would be followed by the establishment of training schools, which would lead directly to the consideration of standards and recognition in the community. The practitioners pushing for prescribed training, and the first ones to go through it, would combine to form a professional association. Wilensky postulated that the next steps would be inter-occupational conflict between the new practitioners and older established occupations in the same sphere, the definition of core tasks, efforts to gain support of the law for areas of practice and the prescription of an ethical code. This sequence was challenged on the grounds that in Britain the formation of professional associations had emerged before the founding of training schools, whether professionally run or university based (Johnson 1972).[5] Nevertheless, having accepted this reordering the pattern put forward by Wilensky, by Carr-Saunders & Wilson, and by Greenwood seems to have been followed in the development of physiotherapy, which stands up as a profession when tested against these criteria. The claims of physiotherapy to full professional status turn largely upon the issue of autonomy and the extent of their freedom from control by the medical profession.

The history and development of physiotherapy as a profession

A review of the development of physiotherapy illustrates the connection with related professions, including medicine. In the 1880s, Swedish remedial gymnasts came to this country and were as Wickstead—historian of the early years of the profession of physiotherapy—writes, freely employed by the progressive members of the medical profession for 'medical rubbing' (Wickstead 1948).[6] This migration of Swedish masseuses led to British women taking up this work as an alternative to, or in addition to, nursing and midwifery. In 1894, an organization called the Society of Trained Masseuses was established by a small group of nurses and midwives dedicated to medical rubbing and determined to protect it from the massage scandals that were common at the time. By 1896 this Society was inviting patronage from eminent doctors and was seeking medical assistance in qualifying its students. Certificates of competence were presented to students when they reached a satisfactory standard. The Society soon contrived a code of conduct for its members and thus at this early stage in its development the Society had accorded with three of the stages in the natural history of professionalization, i.e. the founding of an association based on training, examinations of competence and an ethical code.

In 1900, the name of the Society was changed to the Incorporated Society of Trained Masseuses. Although the medical profession had recognized the Society of Trained Masseuses, the founders realized at an early stage that they had no public or legal status and no legal hold over its members. Therefore, application was made for incorporation under the Companies Act without the use of the word 'limited' as the omission of this word indicated incorporation as a professional and not as a business organization.

In 1905, male nursing orderlies of the Royal Medical Corps were allowed to take the examinations of the Society, but were not at that stage admitted to membership. Male masseurs could not become members as membership carried with it the right to membership of the Trained Nurses Club. Wickstead pointed out that admission of male members to a nurses' social club would, at that time, have created a major scandal.

The establishment of physiotherapy was greatly facilitated by the 1914–18 war, when huge numbers of war wounded, especially amputees, greatly increased the experience of orthopaedic surgeons. Many more patients thus survived disabling injuries and the surgeon looked to the masseuses for rehabilitation work. This increased reliance by the medical profession on trained masseuses, who had extended their range of techniques and treatments to provide a wider range of services, resulted in greater public recognition of the profession.

Recognition was symbolized in 1920 by the granting of the Royal Charter by King George V. This had been preceded in 1916 by the Queen having consented to become Patron of the Society. On the granting of the Royal Charter, the Society changed its name to the Chartered Society of Massage and Medical Gymnastics, and in 1920 men were admitted to membership for the first time.

Between 1920 and 1939, the Chartered Society of Massage and Medical Gymnastics continued to develop as a national organization. A structure of boards and local branches was established throughout the country. Branch constitutions were drawn up and the branches were given financial assistance from Headquarters' funds. By 1929, six local branches had been formed and by 1942 the number had risen to 50 branches. A Branch's Organizer was appointed to the Society Headquarters' staff in 1938.

The Second World War created an increased demand for physiotherapy services and the Armed Forces set up their own physiotherapy schools. A group of male medical gymnasts set up an organization, the Society of Remedial Gymnasts.

The founding of the NHS in 1948 allowed the Chartered Society of Physiotherapy, as it had been known since 1942, to become the dominant occupational group in the remedial therapy services.

The physiotherapy training schools were absorbed into the new NHS, which provided financial security, in contrast to the occupational therapy schools which had been formally organized in the 1930s and whose training schools remained privately funded (Mercer 1978).[7]

In the new NHS, the Chartered Society continued as the qualifying association and professional body, and further developed a centralized and efficient bureaucracy. The tradition of medical patronage remains strong. The decision-making body within the Society, its Council, appointed distinguished doctors as chairmen until 1972 when the first physiotherapist since the granting of the Royal Charter in 1920, Miss Lois E. Dyer, was elected Chairman of Council. In 1920, when the Royal Charter was granted, the Council comprised: 16 elected members of the Society; six honorary members (all founders); eight co-opted members, including seven doctors, and a Baronet. The present list of Council membership is: seven co-opted members (three medical, two lay, one Department of Health Physiotherapy Officer and one other); two student members and 37 physiotherapist members. The Society's policies are now, therefore, decided by physiotherapists within their own organization. This process of slowly evolving autonomy of decision-making accorded with the idea of the development of professionalization on a continuum; movement of occupational groups through a variety of intermediate changes 'culminating in approximation to an "ideal" type of profession' (Goode 1969).[8]

The Chartered Society of Physiotherapy has evolved into a decision-making body with its own ethical code of practice. It controls education for and membership of the profession, and takes action against those members who breach its code of ethics and against unqualified people who claim the title 'Chartered Physiotherapist'.

The establishment of the physiotherapy professional association did not give rise to inter-occupational conflict in the early days. The medical profession retained a firm control over the new Society, the founders having actively sought the patronage of eminent medical men. The ethical code of practice of the profession forbade the treatment of patients, except by direct referral from a doctor. Originally, physiotherapists carried out doctors' instructions much in the same way as a pharmacist would dispense a prescription. During the Society's early decades, the willingness of members to be directed by doctors served to reinforce this practice. The term 'semi-professions' was coined (Etzioni 1969)[9] to identify those would-be professions which exhibited some of the characteristics of the 'ideal' professions. This is an elaboration of the trait method of definition, which comprises a list of attributes which are said to represent the common core of professional occupations. Etzioni suggested that semi-professions were deficient as professions because their training was shorter, their mandate to control their work was less fully granted, their right to privileged communication was less established, there was less of a specialized body of knowledge and less individual autonomy because there was more supervision.

The executive capacity of the Chartered Society of Physiotherapy (CSP), in setting, conducting, examining and awarding its own qualifications, is subject to the approval of the Council for Professions Supplementary to Medicine (CPSM). This was set up by Act of Parliament in 1960, and was welcomed by physiotherapists and the other professions involved. The term 'professions supplementary to medicine' replaced the previously used terms of 'paramedical' and 'medical auxiliary'. The CPSM, through its constituent Boards which were set up as a consequence of the 1960 Act of Parliament, took over the inspection of physiotherapy schools and was responsible for approving any changes which the CSP proposed in curriculum or qualifying procedures.

Each of the member professions of the CPSM was represented by its Board on the Council. Physiotherapy was one of these professions. The Physiotherapists' Board comprised nine elected physiotherapists, six physicians, one educationalist and one physicist. The physiotherapy members, therefore, had a very slender majority on their own Board. All decisions of the Physiotherapists' Board were referred to the Council for ratification and, at this level, the physiotherapy curriculum was lost from total control by physiotherapists. The CPSM had 21 members, the Chairman of the Board together with representatives of the Privy Council and the DHSS. There were three medical representatives from the English Colleges, two doctors representing the Scottish Corporations and one representative of the General Medical Council. When all seats which could be occupied by doctors were so occupied, there would be eight of them. This was a majority as the Professions Supplementary to Medicine were represented by seven members only, only one of whom could be a physiotherapist. The remaining seats were occupied by civil service appointees.

The CPSM was not the end of the decision-making process, but was part of a larger hierarchy. Decisions which had been ratified by the CPSM were submitted to the Privy Council and thence to the Secretary of State, in whom ultimate control was vested. The CPSM structure and procedures remain the same today. Implicit in State Registration, brought about by the setting up of the CPSM under the 1960 Act of Parliament, was the increasing public recognition of physiotherapy; public confidence rests upon the knowledge of maintained standards. It is the responsibility of the CPSM regularly to inspect schools of physiotherapy, and they have the power to enforce changes recommended. Furthermore, any physiotherapist working in the NHS must be registered with the CPSM and have undertaken a training acceptable to that body. '. . . to attain the autonomy of a profession, the paramedical occupation must control a fairly discrete area of work, that can be separated from the main body of medicine and that can be practised without routine contact with or dependence on medicine' (Friedson 1971).[10]

Physiotherapists have an advanced level of clinical autonomy based on clinical diagnosis, although working closely under the umbrella of the doctor's medical diagnosis (see Chapter 3). This contrasts with nursing, more often thought of as a semi-profession, where much of the work is dependent on direction from the doctors.

Measured against the criteria laid down by Carr-Saunders, Friedson, Etzioni and others, a discrete body of knowledge, length of training, formation of an association, ethical codes, community sanction and so on, physiotherapy as an occupational group has moved far along the continuum of professionalization (see Table 2.1 at the conclusion of this chapter).

Physiotherapists work within a specific area of practice and the occupational group has its own distinct history, role, characteristics and relationships with other health professions. The important issue is that this profession, the third largest patient care group in the NHS, has many characteristics which have a significant influence on the way in which the service is managed and provided.

Chartered physiotherapists have a well-developed professional association with selective entry and an ethical code which places constraint and regulation upon its members. Physiotherapy forms a distinctive culture within the Health Service. There is a knowledge, competency and skill base peculiar to the group, and undisputed expertise. There is well-developed clinical and managerial autonomy (see Chapter 3), and acceptance of the clinical role in society, as indicated by the 1960 Professions Supplementary to Medicine Act.

Many of the facets of physiotherapy management discussed throughout this book originate from the professionalization of physiotherapy. An understanding of the professionalization process and what it is that constitutes a profession is crucial to effective and efficient management. Optimum effectiveness and efficiency are, therefore, only achievable through the management of physiotherapy by physiotherapists.

Table 2.1. The process of professionalization—major landmarks

Traits and characteristics	Physiotherapy
1. Formation of an Association	1894—Foundation of Society of Trained Masseuses. Now Chartered Society of Physiotherapy (national organization)
2. Ethical code of practice (standards of conduct)	1895—First ethical code introduced 1987—New rules of professional conduct (ethical code). CSP takes sanction against members who breach ethical code
3. Qualifying examinations and tests of competence	1896—First certificates of competence awarded Present day—three- and four-year degree courses. Steady progress towards all-graduate profession
4. Public, community sanction/recognition	1916—Royal patronage 1920—Royal Charter granted 1960—Professions Supplementary to Medicine Act
5. Discrete body of knowledge and area of practice	1920—Royal Charter enshrines core areas of practice 'massage, medical gymnastics, electrotherapeutics and kindred methods of treatment'
6. Specialized service	Sole occupational group providing physiotherapy. Core tasks, see above
7. Training schools, systematic theory and specialist body of knowledge	35 training schools in the UK. CSP curriculum of study. Wide-ranging physiotherapy literature. Increasing research base. Clinical interest groups
8. Full-time practice	Full-time service provision within NHS and outside it
9. Support of the Law for practice	1960—Professions Supplementary to Medicine Act
10. Autonomy	Well-developed clinical and managerial autonomy, see Chapter 3
11. Autonomy of decision-making	CSP Council
12. Restricted entry	Membership through education and examinations only

3 The Growth of Autonomy in Physiotherapy
R.J. Jones

A well-developed independent status and level of autonomy are important aspects of the professionalization process. Clinical and managerial autonomy embrace complex sets of relationships, and the development of these autonomies has an important influence on the way in which physiotherapy services are managed today. The role of the physiotherapy profession and the provision of service was, for many years, extensively shaped by control over physiotherapy practice by the medical profession. However, over the years there has been a steady and clear move away from this control and self-management has developed, leading to increasing clinical and therapeutic independence.

Background

In the early days of the NHS, the influence of the medical profession in regard to the direction, prescription, training and supervision of physiotherapy, was very powerful. Official Ministry of Health (MoH) memoranda issued in 1949 stated that physiotherapy should be prescribed and directed by a specialist (doctor) (MoH 1949).[1] These views were reinforced in 1951, when the *Report of the Committee on Medical Auxiliaries*, The Cope Report (MoH 1951),[2] was published.

In 1949, a series of eight committees were set up by Aneurin Bevan (Minister of Health). The committees were chaired by Mr. V. Zachary Cope MD MS FRCS, and their membership comprised 'people with Special Experience chosen as individuals and not as representatives of any organization' (MoH 1951).[3]

The brief for the Cope Committee was to report on the supply and demand, training and qualification of certain medical auxiliaries employed in the NHS.

At the time of the Cope Report, physiotherapists, along with seven other occupational groups, were known as medical auxiliaries. The eight sub-committees, one for each occupational group, met separately under the overall co-ordination of Mr. Cope and two Ministry officials. There were no plenary sessions, medical auxiliaries from different occupations being kept separate and always being outnumbered by doctors and Ministry officials. 'The medical auxiliary participants were Ministry nominees, and were not representatives from the Professional Association, which were limited to giving evidence only' (Larkin 1983).[4]

The report reaffirmed that physiotherapists were auxiliaries. Auxiliaries are defined as 'persons who assist medical practitioners (other than as nurses) in the investigation and treatment of disease by virtue of some special skill acquired through a recognized course of training' (MoH 1951).[5] The dominant role of the medical profession was emphasized: 'In every hospital one consultant, preferably a specialist in physical medicine, should be given the oversight of a department . . . to prevent unnecessary work in the physiotherapy department, treatment should be prescribed in all cases by a medical or surgical specialist . . . the general direction of studies in each School should be in the hands of a medical practitioner who should, wherever possible, be a specialist in physical medicine' (MoH 1951).[6]

Doctors were seen as taking the lead in the qualifying examinations of physiotherapists; it was recommended that half of the examiners should be chosen from a panel of medical practitioner examiners. The idea that the auxiliaries should validate their own qualifications was dismissed as unsatisfactory. The reports also recommended that a statutory body be set up to undertake a review of educational standards, and to ensure that the demand for auxiliaries was matched by a well-trained supply. The statutory body envisaged would comprise a two-tier system in which medical auxiliaries would be in a minority on the policy-making council, but would be allowed a majority on the supervisory council. It is clear from this that the medical auxiliaries (including physiotherapists) were officially regarded as being totally subordinate to the medical profession.

The proposals of the Cope Committee were abandoned by the Minister of Health as a result of the occupational groups refusing to co-operate. Following the abandonment of the Cope Report, the Ministry of Health reopened discussion with the medical auxiliaries in 1954. For the first time, each profession was invited to nominate two delegates to the discussions which would encompass the possibility of a method of State Registration.

After years of debate and discussion, the Professions Supplementary to Medicine Bill was introduced into the House of Commons in 1959 and this led to the 1960 Act of Parliament (see Chapter 2) which provided for the registration of eight professions, including physiotherapy. Physiotherapy had won the status of a Profession Supplementary to Medicine under the Act, which provided a statutory framework that allowed for the professions to regulate themselves for the protection of their patients.

At this time, the staffing structure in a physiotherapy department was, typically, a Superintendent Physiotherapist, senior physiotherapists and basic-grade staff. In some parts of the country, there were Group Superintendents who acted as Head Physiotherapists for several hospitals.

Physiotherapy was mostly based in general hospitals with minimal input to community, mental illness, special needs or special schools. The role of the Superintendent was originally that of clinical leader of the department. Gradually, the duties expanded to include administrative responsibilities.

In 1972, the Tunbridge Report (DHSS 1972)[7] was published. The brief of the Tunbridge Committee had been 'to consider the future provision of rehabilitation services in the National Health Service, their organization and development, and to make recommendations'.

The members of the Tunbridge Committee were all doctors. There was no representation from the remedial professions (at that time, physiotherapy, remedial gymnastics and occupational therapy were known collectively as the remedial professions). The Tunbridge Committee worked in association with the Committee on the Remedial Professions, which had been appointed in 1969 by the Secretary of State for Social Services and the Secretaries of State for Scotland and Wales. The remit of the Committee on the Remedial Professions was 'To consider the function and inter-relationship of occupational therapists, physiotherapists and remedial gymnasts in the National Health Service, their relation to other personnel concerned with rehabilitation and the broad pattern of staff required, and to make recommendations' (DHSS 1972).[8] In order to maintain close liaison between the two committees, four members of the Tunbridge Committee were also members of the Committee on the Remedial Professions. Written and oral evidence was gathered by the Tunbridge Committee and visits were made by its members to a number of establishments which provided various forms of rehabilitation.

Physiotherapists were very disappointed by the recommendations of the Tunbridge Committee. The report served only to reinforce the old dogma emphasizing the dominance of the medical profession in the management, supervision and clinical role of physiotherapy. There were many statements throughout the entire report which argued for the continued dominance by the medical profession, for example, on the question of how rehabilitation departments should be organized and who should be in charge of them. 'The consultant will have overall managerial responsibility for the rehabilitation services, and will decide how the general day-to-day running of the rehabilitation department should be organized according to local circumstances . . . We recommend that delegation of responsibility for day-to-day treatment of patients should be permitted to members of the remedial professions, provided that they are always under the supervision of the appropriate consultant' (DHSS 1972).[9]

The consultant in rehabilitation (with responsibility for remedial services) was to be responsible for planning the general programmes of rehabilitation for patients, organizing facilities for the assessment of social, vocational and clinical aspects of disability, and the reasonable deployment of all remedial staff from the most senior therapist to aide.

It is clear, therefore, that physiotherapists were regarded by the Tunbridge Committee as technicians to be totally organized, managed and clinically supervised by consultant medical staff. Physiotherapists would have little, if any, managerial responsibility for even the day-to-day running of the departments in which they worked. Their clinical practice would be totally dictated by the prescriptions laid down by consultants, who were to be in a position of complete control of rehabilitation services, even as far as physiotherapy techniques and everyday practice were concerned. This would be reflected in a system of training whereby physiotherapy students would be taught only those techniques and practices likely to be prescribed by the consultants, however inappropriate such methods might have been. As a result, there would be no encouragement of research and evaluation of practice; the physiotherapists would assume the role of 'handmaidens' to the medical profession.

So disappointed were the representatives from the remedial professions that they refused to endorse the report and instead wrote their own *Statement by the Committee on the Remedial Professions* (DHSS 1972).[10] The statement expressed the need for the provision of representation from the remedial professions on advisory committees at both regional and area levels, so as to ensure participation in policy formulation and decision making as these affected their activities. The need for research into the treatments and techniques employed by the remedial professions was acknowledged, as were the differing roles of the three remedial professions. The role of the Domiciliary Therapist was emphasized and the setting up of a career structure in which there were more senior posts with clinical, research and teaching responsibilities was recommended. The Tunbridge Report had restated old ideas on the dominance of the medical profession over physiotherapy. The statement, while recognizing some aspects of this, had made positive recommendations on representation, research, career structure, domiciliary therapy and the opportunity for therapists to decide on the application and duration of treatments. If these recommendations were accepted, a further step towards autonomy would have been achieved. The remedial professions, through their committee representatives, played a key role in the production of the statement, which would not have been published without sustained pressure from them (Patrick 1986).[11]

Genesis of District physiotherapy management posts

A watershed in professional independence

As a result of the disquiet caused by the Tunbridge Report, a Working Party, under the chairmanship of Mr. E. L. McMillan, was set up in 1973 by Sir Keith Joseph, the Secretary of State for Social Services. It was to make recommendations on the future role of the remedial professions in relation to 'other professions and to the patient, and on the pattern of staffing and training needed to meet this' (DHSS 1973).[12] The Working Party comprised one senior member of each of the three remedial professions (physiotherapy, occupational therapy and remedial gymnastics), a representative from the CPSM, and four members from the DHSS. The Scottish Home and Health Department was represented at the meetings by an observer. The problem areas considered by the Working Party included:

- misuse and waste of professional skills;
- dissatisfaction with career and salary structure;
- shortage of trained therapists;
- inadequate support from clerical, secretarial and portering staff;
- problems of overlapping of responsibilities, not only between the remedial professions themselves, but also between them and other professions.

The Working Party recognized that in NHS hospitals the remedial professions had very limited managerial responsibilities associated with their clinical duties. These professions were often represented at management and policy-making levels by nursing or medical colleagues. McMillan acknowledged that senior members of the remedial professions 'may organize their own departments though often this is within a framework set by a consultant' (DHSS 1973).[13]

On the relationship between the remedial professions and the medical profession, the McMillan Report acknowledged the doctor as the 'key figure' in carrying primary clinical responsibility for the patient; however, the report spelled out clearly the Working Party's concern that frequently this was interpreted as requiring the doctor to prescribe and supervise in detail the therapy provided by the remedial professions. In criticizing these practices, the report noted that too often 'therapists' are given insufficient scope to exercise their skills to the best possible advantage of the patient (DHSS 1973).[14] McMillan drew attention to the scarce opportunities for members of the remedial professions to take on managerial roles or to receive appropriate management training.

The McMillan recommendations would profoundly affect the development of clinical relationships between the physiotherapy and medical professions, as well as the organization and management of physiotherapy services. The report stated: 'Few doctors who refer patients will be skilled in the detailed application by therapists of particular techniques, although there will be exceptions. With this in mind, it should surely be possible for the doctor and therapists to work together in an atmosphere of mutual respect and appreciation . . . we attach the greatest importance to this relationship. We think it follows that the therapist can operate more effectively only if given greater responsibility and freedom within a medically orientated team . . .' (DHSS 1973).[15] McMillan also recommended that the nature and duration of treatment should be for the therapist to determine. An important recommendation in the report about the management and organization of the remedial professions was that they should co-ordinate, organize and administer their own services. This was 'in keeping with the principle that professional people are more properly managed by members of their own profession' (DHSS 1973).[16]

Furthermore, this approach was strengthened by the recommendation that there should be a therapist at District level with management responsibilities for hospital and community remedial services. These bold recommendations marked a watershed in the development of the physiotherapy service. It was the first time that such recommendations had appeared in an official report or Government document and would pave the way, together with the other recommendations, for the development of self-management and clinical responsibility in the remedial professions. The McMillan Report was clearly a quantum leap from the recommendations contained in the Tunbridge Report, and the plethora of reports and circulars published earlier.

The 1974 NHS reorganization and beyond

In August 1972, the Government published a White Paper entitled *National Health Service Reorganization: England* which led to the National Health Service Reorganization Bill in November 1972 (DHSS 1972).[17] The consequent National Health Service Reorganization Act was given Royal Assent on 5 July 1973 (25 years to the day after the NHS came into existence).

The *Management Arrangements for the Reorganized National Health Service*, the Grey Book (DHSS 1972),[18] was published towards the end of that year, shortly after the Government White Paper. This document described the Regional and Area Health Authorities (RHAs and AHAs) and their functions, and outlined job descriptions for some of the new posts at all levels of the organization.

The Grey Book contained a chapter concerning paramedical work and the arrangements for physiotherapy were briefly outlined in it. In the introduction to this chapter *Paramedical Work* (DHSS 1972),[19] it was stated: 'The paramedical services have been organized mainly in very small sections and departments within the hospital service, and, in some few cases, within the local authority health service. Most of these services however, will be organized on a district basis, to be available both within hospitals and to medical practice outside hospitals . . .' (DHSS 1972).[20]

Physiotherapy would be accountable to a Consultant in Physical Medicine or a direct appointee of the AHA. A senior physiotherapist, such as a Superintendent, could be appointed as the professional head of service, and would be monitored by the District Administrator and also by the consultants and general practitioners 'prescribing' the service for their patients.

It was recommended that as part of the monitoring process, the District Management Team (DMT) would carry out a systematic review of all the services of the professions supplementary to medicine. The Grey Book envisaged the appointment of an Area Convenor whose role would be to ensure that professional and technical standards were being maintained, and would negotiate temporary inter-District loans of personnel, to cope with serious local shortages. The Area Convenor was to be one of the District heads of the professions supplementary to medicine.

It was the purpose of the Grey Book to make recommendations on management, and arrangements for the reorganization, and many of the proposals it contained were significant for the development of physiotherapy services. Although total managerial independence for physiotherapy was not proposed, the need for a professional head of service on a District-wide basis was recognized. Furthermore, it would be possible under the provisions of the Grey Book for the professional head of service, in conjunction with consultant medical staff, to give advice to the DMT. One radical proposal concerned accountability; the head of physiotherapy services could be accountable either to the Consultant in Physical Medicine, or to the District Administrator. It was proposed, for the first time, that accountability for physiotherapy services could rest outside the medical profession. These recommendations were much less radical for the organization of the service than those contained in the McMillan Report (which had focused on the remedial professions only). However, it is significant that some of the ideas are common to both documents. In its acceptance of the concept of a physiotherapy service organized on a District basis, a professional head of service from within physiotherapy itself, and the possibility of advising the DMT, the Grey Book was part of the general trend towards the strengthening of physiotherapy autonomy. Some of the proposals were not implemented, but the Grey Book clearly represented a further stage in the gradual change of official thinking. The proposals could be altered after consultation. However, very little time was allowed for the consultation process as the legislation to introduce reorganization was to come into force on 1 April 1974.

By 1974, most hospital management committees had Group Superintendent Physiotherapists who assumed more general responsibilities for physiotherapy, both in terms of effective resource management and for ensuring the professional quality of the service. Before the 1974 NHS reorganization, when there were hospital groups and group secretaries, there had been many problems for physiotherapy services. Staff could be recruited to the large acute hospitals whereas small hospitals and geriatric units, for example, could not attract them. This problem was eased, to some extent, by making the Senior Superintendent Physiotherapist the group head of service. The Group Superintendent also took responsibility for developing community physiotherapy services and, in a few cases, general practitioner open access to physiotherapy departments. The Group Superintendent posts were not officially recognized; there was no Whitley Council pay scale for them. However, authorities gradually accepted that it was necessary for someone to carry out these and other tasks of co-ordination and management.

A health circular, *The Remedial Professions and Linked Therapies* HSC(IS)101 (DHSS 1974),[21] was published giving guidance to health authorities on the interim arrangements for the organization of the services of the remedial professions and linked therapies (industrial, art, drama and music therapy). The guidance in this health circular was intended to be effective for at least 18 months while discussions between the DHSS, the remedial professions and other organizations concerned with the future structure of the remedial professions, took place in the light of the McMillan Report.

A foundation for the possible development of District Physiotherapist appointments was laid down by this health circular: 'Services will normally be organized on a District basis, either separately or partially grouped (e.g. combined physiotherapy – remedial gymnast departments), or in a comprehensive department of rehabilitation . . . the Area Health Authority should designate in Districts a Senior Physiotherapist . . . as having responsibility for advising management teams. These therapists, in conjunction with medical advice, will advise District Community Physicians on the organization of their services for the District and will be responsible for ensuring that professional standards are maintained' (DHSS 1974).[22]

It was not intended that these therapists should relinquish all of their clinical duties; however, health authorities were reminded that there would be a diminution of the clinical duties that such a 'designated' therapist would be expected to undertake. The health circular recommended that the designated therapist was to be accountable to the District Community Physician for the special new responsibilities. It was recognized that post-holders would require administrative support which would be made available by the District or Area Administrators. Furthermore, on the question of advice to AHAs and RHAs on matters affecting the remedial professions, this document recommended that these authorities should obtain advice from the professions concerned. All of these recommendations formed the most positive step yet towards the introduction of District Therapist appointments, and were an important move towards managerial autonomy.

The structure of the pay and conditions of service for physiotherapists and the other professions supplementary to medicine was established in 1975 with the publication of the *Report of the Committee of Inquiry into the pay and related conditions of service of the Professions Supplementary to Medicine and Speech Therapists*—Halsbury Report (DHSS 1975).[23] This committee, chaired by Lord Halsbury, radically revised the grading structure for these professions. As a result, there would be a basic grade for newly qualified staff, two grades of Senior Physiotherapist and four grades of

Superintendent. The post of District Physiotherapist was also mentioned, but not discussed further because these posts were not yet fully developed.

The Government's adoption of the Halsbury Report meant that the total grading structure of physiotherapy was expanded, widening the scope for clinical specialization, research and management, resulting in a profession which was more complex and wide ranging. The Senior 1 grade, for example, would allow experienced staff to become more involved in specialized areas such as manipulative therapy, community domiciliary physiotherapy, paediatrics, respiratory and intensive care, mental illness, care of amputees and others. These new opportunities meant that there was an increased need to organize and manage the service in a co-ordinated way in order to prevent fragmentation of services and resources, and facilitate the most effective use of scarce clinical expertise. It became increasingly necessary for the service to be managed at District level.

An agreement on remuneration, which allowed payment of an allowance to designated District therapists, was published in Advance Letter (PTA) 20/75 (DHSS 1975).[24] This was a further advance in the development of District physiotherapy posts. The success of these negotiations showed that the DHSS (management side of the Whitley Council) had accepted the need for such posts and was willing to make payment for the work undertaken by designated District Therapists. The DHSS also circulated clear recommendations on the job description and procedures for such appointments in DS331/75 (DHSS 1975).[25]

In 1977, the *Report of the Sub-group on the Organization of the Remedial Professions in the National Health Service* (DHSS 1977)[26] was published. This sub-group had been established by the DHSS co-ordinating committee on the implementation of the McMillan Report and comprised representatives from the DHSS, the three remedial professions, District physicians, members of the British Association of Rheumatology and Rehabilitation, and a chairman. Its purpose was to consider how a future management structure could be developed for the remedial professions from the existing interim arrangements.

In the view of the sub-group, there were weaknesses in previously published Department of Health advice and they recommended that in order to maintain the most effective use and deployment of remedial services within a District, each of the three professions would need to be organized at District level. Managerial, administrative and advisory tasks were identified, and it was also noted that remedial services were necessary within all client groups and 'most specialities' throughout the NHS.

However, the report did not suggest a single solution for all health Districts, accepting that needs varied according to differing circumstances in different Districts. The objective of undertaking managerial tasks was recognized as being ultimately to improve the standard of care to the people they served, and it was also noted that the remedial therapies should be seen in perspective as part of the far wider rehabilitation services.

The role of consultants and other professional groups concerned was recognized. There would need to be extensive and continuous collaboration between them and the remedial professions in order to facilitate effective management.

The major recommendation of the report was that Districts should appoint District Therapists in physiotherapy, occupational therapy and remedial gymnastics to manage, organize and plan their services, and that District planning procedures were to include the District Therapists' input.

A health circular, *Health Services Development, Management of the Remedial Professions in the NHS* HC(79)19 (DHSS 1979)[27] was published following its issue the previous year as a draft circular for consultation. The draft, not numbered or dated, invited comments from interested parties. Broadly, the findings of this draft reiterated those of the sub-group: 'The Department, however, is in no doubt that the professions should be managed by themselves, and believes that the arguments and recommendations in the report . . . now provide the best and most logical way forward' (DHSS 1978).[28]

Five years had elapsed since the publication of the McMillan Report when the DHSS issued this unequivocal statement. However, the draft circular only advised to Health Authorities; it did not lay down specific instructions for authorities. It recommended that as soon as resources allowed, health authorities appoint District Therapists to manage and plan the services of their professions.

The District Therapists were to be accountable to a DMT member and, for clinical matters, it was recommended that HC(77)33 be adhered to (*see* below). The post of District Physiotherapist was, therefore, finally constituted to manage and plan physiotherapy services on a District-wide basis. Many Health Authorities proceeded to make District appointments, and many of those authorities which had previously employed a designated District Physiotherapist made the post substantive. Approximately 160 of the Districts in England and Wales had made District Physiotherapist appointments by the time that the Griffiths Report was published in 1983 (Jones 1987)[29] which showed that physiotherapists had achieved a substantial degree of managerial autonomy.

Clinical autonomy

An important development in the practice of physiotherapy during recent years has been the growing recognition of the rights of Chartered Physiotherapists in clinical differential diagnosis and the control of therapy. The DHSS issued a code of practice in September 1977, *Health Services Development—Relationship between the Medical and Remedial Professions*

HC(77)33 (DHSS 1977).[30] This important document recognized the right of physiotherapists to make their own decisions on prescribing appropriate forms of physiotherapy treatment for patients referred by medical practitioners; therefore, the referral by a doctor could be as open as 'physiotherapy please'. This document also gave formal recognition to the right of physiotherapists to alter or terminate treatment, if appropriate in their professional judgment. If a physiotherapist were to accept detailed prescriptions of treatment from doctors (such as short-wave diathermy twice a week), rather than a note of the medical diagnosis, reason for referral and information concerning relevant contraindications, that therapist was accepting the doctor's knowledge of physiotherapy practice as being greater than his/her own.

However the doctor, in referring patients for physiotherapy, was not seen as handing over total control but, in asking for treatment by a therapist, was asking for the help of another qualified professional.

The circular also stated that the therapist had a duty and a consequential right to decline to perform any therapy which his/her professional training and expertise suggested was actively harmful to the patient.

In HC(77)33, there was a statement by the Standing Medical Advisory Committee on the relationship between the medical and remedial professions, '. . . in the context of the NHS the relationship between the doctors and therapists (both in hospitals of all types and in the community) has been developed by convention guided by the Codes of Practice set out by the statutory and professional bodies of the therapists concerned. Therapists are in very close contact with their patients during treatment and therefore develop the facility for equating the different forms of treatment to the pattern of patient response. More use should be made of this experience . . .' (DHSS 1977).[31]

The observations and recommendations of this health circular and the accompanying statement were a long way removed from those of the Tunbridge Report. As a document concerning the respective roles of doctors and physiotherapists, HC(77)33 was an important landmark.

The McMillan Report, which had resulted from sustained pressure by the remedial professions, had foreshadowed much of the contents of HC(77)33. The circular represented a further step in the developing independence and responsibility of physiotherapists, both by its recognition of current practice and by making positive recommendations concerning future relationships. The level of clinical autonomy for physiotherapists, which the circular recognized and protected, followed on from the developments taking place in the management and organization of physiotherapy services in the NHS.

Towards the 1982 NHS reorganization

The Royal Commission on the NHS, Merrison Report (Royal Commission 1979),[32] reported on 18 July 1979, following the election of a new Conservative Government in May of that year, under the premiership of

Mrs Margaret Thatcher. The Royal Commission had been set up by the previous Labour Government and had taken three years to complete its task. Its main conclusion was that 'we need not be ashamed of our health service and that there are many aspects of it of which we can be justly proud'. However, it was critical of some aspects of NHS management, for example, too many management tiers, too many administrators, a slow decision-making process and a consequent waste of money.

In December, a consultative document *Patients First* (DHSS 1979)[33] was published as the new Government's response to the Royal Commission Report. *Patients First* aimed to simplify the organizational structure of the NHS and to incorporate some of its recommendations. It was the philosophy of *Patients First* to move responsibility for making decisions closer to the locality for which services were being provided. The AHAs were seen as being remote from the local service providers, the patients and the local community. A major recommendation was that the District should become the key accountable body in the new structure, being responsible for planning and for service provision. The arrangement of DHAs in the NHS, until the advent of the Government White Paper *Working for Patients*, derives largely from the recommendations of this consultative document and the DHSS Circular, *Health Services Development Structure and Management* HC(80)8 (DHSS 1980)[34] which followed. This endorsed:

- the removal of the Area tier of management;
- that decisions should be taken as near to the patient as possible;
- that the professional consultative machinery should be simplified and unit management based on hospitals should be introduced.

These policies were later embodied in the 1982 NHS reorganization. At the same time, the DHSS attached a specific salary scale to the post of District Physiotherapist and indicated how the various grades were to be banded into District I, II and III. By placing a financial value on substantive posts, the Department was clearly supporting the concept of a self-managed profession at District level.

Advice relevant to District appointments was issued in HC(80)8. 'When considering management accountability of officers, Authorities should assure themselves that a manager can appropriately be held accountable for the work of a particular individual. This is especially relevant when considering whether a member of the administrative disciplines can be made managerially accountable for non-administrative staff' (DHSS 1980).[35] This instruction reinforced the idea of professional staff being managed by members of their own profession.

Ethical code

Ethical matters are of considerable concern to health care professionals, including physiotherapists. An important function of the Chartered Society of Physiotherapy (CSP) is to maintain high ethical standards, as embodied in its Rules of Professional Conduct (CSP 1986).[36] The ethical code of practice aims to protect the public (patients and clients of physiotherapists) from professional malpractice and misconduct. 'To the layman the word "Ethics" suggests a set of standards by which a particular group or community decides to regulate its behaviour—to distinguish what is legitimate or acceptable in pursuit of their aims from what is not' (Flew 1979).[37]

The former rules, which had been approved by the Privy Council in 1978, were largely prescriptive, leaving little room for individual practitioners to exercise professional judgment. The final proposals on the new Rules of Professional Conduct were unanimously accepted by CSP Council in the December of 1984 and were published in *Physiotherapy* April 1986, coming into force with the appropriate Privy Council approval on 1 January 1987.

The new rules were designed to reflect current practice and are not examined in detail here, but some important concepts which underlie them are discussed.

Clinical diagnosis

An integral part of physiotherapy practice – clinical diagnosis – is a rigorous method of history taking, clinical examination and functional assessment. Clinical diagnosis allows conclusions to be drawn concerning possible causes of the patient's problems, enabling appropriate physiotherapy intervention, if any. This emphasizes the problem-solving approach of modern physiotherapy practice. The term clinical diagnosis is used rather than medical or pathological diagnosis. Medical diagnosis (the doctor's prerogative) encompasses clinical diagnosis together with medical test findings, X-rays, biopsies, etc., while pathological diagnosis can only be made at post-mortem examination. The concept of clinical diagnosis underlies the clinical independence of the physiotherapist in deciding appropriate action to be taken, if any. Although the doctor may give a medical diagnosis, the Chartered Physiotherapist's independent professional role is acknowledged. This represents an important marker of physiotherapy autonomy, recognizing the physiotherapist's distinct contribution to patient care within a discrete body of knowledge and skill.

The physiotherapist carries legal responsibility for his/her practice. A doctor's signature on a piece of paper does not offer any immunity from legal proceedings in the event of malpractice (*see* Chapter 6); such a signature does not protect the therapist, who must act in accordance with his/her own professional judgment. When a person is seen by a physiotherapist without an initial referral from a medical practitioner, the physiotherapist has a clear responsibility to liaise with the patient's doctor.

Patients are referred to Chartered Physiotherapists by health care professionals other than doctors, for example, speech therapists and District nurses, as well as from other sources, including self-referrals, social services departments and local education authorities. In all such instances, the physiotherapist has a duty to liaise with the patient's doctor. Physiotherapists also undertake a significant workload which is not the subject of referral; this includes health education and promotion in, for example, ergonomic and postural advice, lifting training and keep fit.

The *modus operandi* and the scope and spectrum of modern physiotherapy practice, as reflected by the Rules of Professional Conduct, are further important markers of the advanced level of autonomy and independence achieved by Chartered Physiotherapists.

Physiotherapy autonomy and the Government White Paper *Working for Patients*

The Government review of the NHS, chaired by the Prime Minister, was completed with the publication (early in 1989) of the White Paper *Working for Patients* (DHSS 1989)[38] (*see* Chapter 5). On 25 September that year, representatives of the CSP met with the Health Minister, David Mellor, at the Department of Health to discuss aspects of the White Paper in relation to physiotherapy practice in the NHS. A paper *Note of Meeting with David Mellor, Minister of State for Health* (CSP 1989)[39] was subsequently published.

The Minister accepted that physiotherapists have the right to make their own assessments and treatment plans, and that this will remain their responsibility. The Government's policy would be to maintain the clinical autonomy of physiotherapy. The White Paper 'did not intend to stop professions evolving effective methods of practice' and he accepted that clinical autonomy for physiotherapists 'was an effective method of practice' (CSP 1989).[40] In May 1990, a further meeting took place between representatives of the Professions Allied to Medicine and David Mellor's successor as Minister for Health, Virginia Bottomley. At this meeting, Mrs Bottomley gave assurances that open referral systems to physiotherapy, including self-referral and inter-professional cross-referral, would be continued in the Health Service under the NHS reforms.

Clearly, therefore, the Government's stated policy is to maintain professional autonomy within physiotherapy.

Relationships between physiotherapy, the medical profession and NHS management have radically changed since the inception of the NHS in 1948. During this period, physiotherapy has achieved managerial and clinical autonomy; Chartered Physiotherapists control their own practice based on professional standards and judgement. Their practice is not circumscribed by a need to appeal to a different or higher authority in physiotherapy practice; there is no higher authority to which such appeals could be made in this context. The question of what therapy, if any, to administer, is concentrated in the hands of physiotherapists themselves and supervision of junior staff is carried out by more experienced physiotherapists.

Clinical autonomy in physiotherapy is dependent upon its managerial autonomy. Inevitably, the clinical independence achieved during the past 40 years would be seriously eroded or lost if the profession were again managed by non-physiotherapists. Management decisions in physiotherapy relate to clinical service and practice.

The NHS is a multi-disciplinary, complex organization and although physiotherapy is an independent clinical profession, it is essential that it be managed in the context of the Health Service as a whole. Integrated and well co-ordinated service provision is necessary for high-quality patient care.

4 General Management
R.J. Jones

General management was introduced into the NHS following the publication of the *National Health Service Management Inquiry*—Griffiths Report—(Griffiths 1983)[1] and the subsequent Department of Health and Social Security (DHSS) Circular HC(84)13, *Health Services Management Implementation of the NHS Management Inquiry Report* (DHSS 1984).[2] The Government decision to implement general management throughout the NHS meant that health authorities were required to bring about changes in their management structures. Therefore, to comply with this policy, it was necessary for DHAs to review their management arrangements, including the organization and management of clinical services such as physiotherapy.

Setting up the NHS management inquiry

For several years, the Government had been dissatisfied with consensus management in the NHS—management by agreement—and less than a year after the 1982 reorganization the NHS management inquiry was set up. In the House of Commons, Mrs Knight asked the Secretary of State for Social Services (Mr Norman Fowler) 'If he will make a statement on his plans to control manpower in the National Health Service' (Hansard 3.2.1983).[3] Norman Fowler's reply to this written question was: 'I have today established an independent NHS management inquiry into these matters. Health Authorities in England have a revenue budget of almost £9 billion; employ about a million people; and spend almost 75 per cent of their revenue on pay. The Government needs to be satisfied that these considerable resources are managed efficiently and give the nation value for money. The inquiry will be led by Sir Roy Griffiths, Deputy Chairman and Managing Director of J Sainsbury PLC . . .'.

Sir Roy Griffiths, in his letter to the Secretary of State attached to his NHS Management Inquiry Report, stated: 'We were asked by you in February to give advice on the effective use and management of manpower and related resources in the National Health Service; to inform you as our inquiries proceeded; and to advise you on progress by the end of June . . . It was emphasized that we had not been asked to prepare a report, but that we should go straight for recommendations on management action' (Griffiths 1983).[4]

This request by the Secretary of State was to prepare the way for a most radical and innovative series of changes in the management and organizational structure of the NHS.

Sir Roy Griffiths and the inquiry team

The Griffiths team comprised members who were experienced in business management rather than health care. Sir Roy Griffiths, Chairman of the Inquiry, was Managing Director of the Sainsbury's Food Chain, Michael Bett was Personnel Director of British Telecom, Jim Blyth was Head of Defence Sales at the Ministry of Defence and Sir Brian Bailey, Chairman of Television South West.

The Inquiry philosophy was clearly influenced by the business background of the team members. Griffiths observed that his team were brought in to advise on the NHS not because they were instant experts on all aspects of the NHS, but because of their business experience. They had been told that the NHS was different from business in management terms, not least because it was not concerned with the profit motive and must be judged by wider social standards which could not be measured. These differences, he claimed, could be greatly overstated.

The Griffiths Inquiry was unique in the history of official investigations into the workings and management of the NHS. The team comprised only four members and there were no medical interests represented, in contrast with the many bodies which had previously reported to successive Secretaries of State on various aspects of the NHS. The Report *Management Arrangements for the Reorganized National Health Service*—the Grey Book—(DHSS 1972)[5] and *Rehabilitation Report of a Sub-committee of the Standing Medical Advisory Committee*—Tunbridge Report—(DHSS 1972)[6] are just two examples where the committees were large (both having more than 15 members), a substantial number were from the medical profession, nursing, other professional interests and the DHSS. However, the membership of the Griffiths team was not the only feature which made the inquiry unique.

Findings and style of the Griffiths Inquiry

The report concluded that there was a lack of drive in the NHS because at each level of management there was no one person held accountable for action; decisions were delayed or avoided, leading to an inefficient service. The main findings of the team were that there was no real continuous evaluation of performance, precise management objectives were rarely set, little measurement of health care output took place, and clinical and economic evaluation of practices was uncommon. One of the most important observations was the identification that a clearly defined general management function was absent from the service. A telling passage from the report simplistically sums this up; 'if Florence Nightingale were carrying her lamp through the corridors of the NHS today she would almost certainly be searching for the people in charge' (Griffiths 1983).[7]

In the section of the report entitled 'general observations', Griffiths outlined in detail the advantages of the general management process. In its advocacy of general management, the team was damning of functional management in that the advantages of the functional specialities were offset by the need to establish the general management process effectively. Consensus management methods were vigorously criticized as being responsible for the making of 'lowest common denominator decisions' which were weak and of poor quality. NHS management was thought to be reactive and passive rather than proactive, and there was a lack of management data on consumer views. Therefore, most of the report was about changes which were needed in attitude, understanding and expectations, as well as the style of management.

The characteristic style of the Griffiths Report is striking in many ways. The team of businessmen brought their own experience and perceptions as managers from outside the Health Service to analyse the way the NHS was run. The report was produced in a very short time (approximately seven months) and, possibly due to this and the backgrounds of the Griffiths team members, was impressionistic, presenting a minimum of factual information, and there was very little reasoning or explanation to support the diagnoses reached. Another important way in which the Griffiths critique of management in the NHS differed from other reports was the absence of any analysis or discussion of previous reports or documents; this led to the tendency for a prescription of instant remedies to NHS ills and a lack of sensitivity to the differences between the roles and functions of business and the Health Service. The Griffiths Report was an innovation in findings, style, structure and team membership, and recommendations were to have a radical and fundamental effect on the organization and structure of the NHS.

Inquiry recommendations

The Secretary of State was advised by Griffiths that he should set up a Health Service Supervisory Board and a full-time NHS Management Board. The Health Service Supervisory Board would be responsible for determining the objectives and direction for the Service, approving overall budget and resource allocations, making strategic decisions and monitoring performance; the Secretary of State would chair the board.

The Management Board would be the executive arm of the Supervisory Board and would have responsibility: 'to plan implementation of the policies approved by the Supervisory Board; to give leadership to the management of the NHS; to control performance; and to achieve consistency and drive over the long term' (Griffiths 1983).[8]

The recommendation to set up the NHS Management Board was a totally new departure in the organization of the Service and would be crucial to the implementation of general management. 'Provided that there is an effective Management Board, including a Director General of substance, one of the Board's key tasks in its early years will be to develop the general management strand at all levels in the NHS. Without that sustained commitment, there is simply no chance that the revolution that Griffiths seeks will take place' (Evans and Maxwell 1983).[9] Below Management Board level, Griffiths advised that the appointment of General Managers should be made at RHA, DHA and Unit levels. These posts would carry responsibility for improving the efficiency of the organization and the appointments could be made either from within the NHS or from outside it. General Managers could, therefore, come from any discipline.

RHA and DHA Chairmen were to be given greater freedom to organize the management structure of the Authorities in the ways best suited to local requirements and management potential. Furthermore, it was recommended that Regional and District Chairmen should review and reduce the need for functional management structures. The primary reporting relationship of functional managers was to be the General Manager. Health Authorities were recommended to initiate major cost improvement programmes for implementation by General Managers. Responsibility for making decisions was to be moved closer to the locality for which services were being provided; in this, the Units would play a key role. All day-to-day decisions were to be taken in the main hospitals and other Units of Management. Each Unit of Management would be given a total budget and would develop *management budgets* which would involve doctors who would be expected to relate workload and service objectives to financial and manpower allocations, in order to 'sharpen up the questioning of overhead costs' (Griffiths 1983).[10]

The report also contained recommendations on personnel, manpower, conditions of service and levels of decision making, which were followed by 14 pages of general observations. Figure 4.1 shows the NHS management structure before the implementation of the Griffiths Report and Figure 4.2 shows the structure as proposed by Griffiths.

Griffiths proposals and Government decisions

In June 1984, HC(84)13 was issued by the DHSS, implementing the Griffiths proposals. The Secretary of State had allowed only a short period of time for consultation on the Inquiry Report (approximately three months);

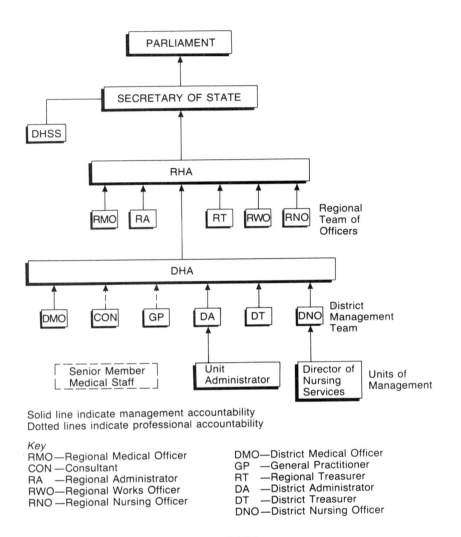

Solid line indicate management accountability
Dotted lines indicate professional accountability

Key
RMO—Regional Medical Officer
CON —Consultant
RA   —Regional Administrator
RWO—Regional Works Officer
RNO —Regional Nursing Officer

DMO—District Medical Officer
GP   —General Practitioner
RT   —Regional Treasurer
DA   —District Administrator
DT   —District Treasurer
DNO—District Nursing Officer

Figure 4.1. NHS management structure pre Griffiths

written comments on the proposals had to be submitted to the DHSS by 9 January 1984.

This health circular reiterated the Griffiths sentiment that the NHS exists to deliver services to people and not to organize systems for their own sake.

Under the provisions of this health circular, the Health Authorities were charged with the task of establishing the general management function and

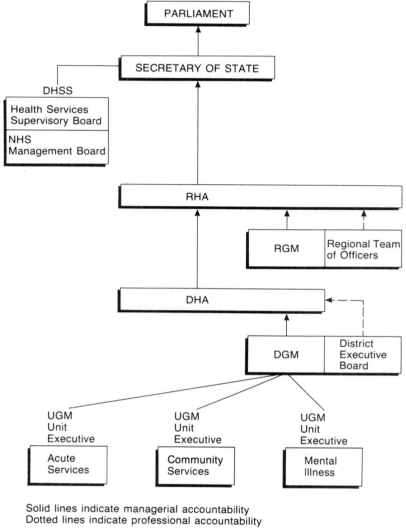

Solid lines indicate managerial accountability
Dotted lines indicate professional accountability

Key
RHA—Regional Health Authority   DGM—District General Manager
DHA—District Health Authority   UGM—Unit General Manager
RGM—Regional General Manager

Figure 4.2. NHS management structure (Griffiths recommendations)

identifying General Managers, and many of the Griffiths Report's recommendations and general observations were to be brought in as policy.
Decisions on the organizational structures were to be left to each Health
Authority. It was emphasized in the health circular that Authorities should
be allowed the maximum flexibility in making their own management
arrangements. This would obviously include management arrangements for
physiotherapy services.

Implementation of the Griffiths Inquiry created a radical and far-reaching
culture change in the organization and management of the Service, despite
the Griffiths team's view that the NHS was in no condition to undergo
another restructuring. The Royal Commission on the NHS—Merrison
Report—(Royal Commission 1979),[11] while making recommendations for
reform, had also expressed the plea that there should be no more major
upheavals in order to enable the NHS to settle down following the 1974
reorganization. However, despite this, the reorganization which took place
in 1982 brought about major changes in the senior administrative levels
of the Service and were followed two years later by the implementation of the
Griffiths recommendations. These, in turn, laid the foundation for the
Government White Paper *Working for Patients* published in 1989, the consequent Health Service Bill enacted in 1990 and the Resource Management
Initiative.

General management

General management was defined by Griffiths as: 'The responsibility drawn
together in one person, at different levels of the organization, for planning,
implementation and control of performance . . .' (Griffiths 1983).[12]

He claimed that the advantages of a general management process were:

- providing the necessary leadership to capitalize on existing high levels
  of dedication and expertise;
- bringing about a constant search for major change and cost
  improvement;
- securing proper motivation of staff;
- ensuring that the professional functions are effectively geared towards
  the overall objectives and responsibilities of the general management
  process;
- making sense of the process of consultation.

As well as vigorously criticizing functional management, the Inquiry team
were scathing about consensus management methods as being responsible
for long delays in the management process.

A General Manager is defined as: 'A manager who determines and
influences the broad objectives of a whole organization, determines the

resources to be made available for attaining those objectives and has significant responsibilities in more than one major field of activity (usually working through managers who specialize in single fields of activity). A General Manager is especially concerned with formulation and interpretation of policy and with long term planning' (French and Saward 1984).[13]

With the introduction of this form of management into the NHS, it was likely that a more authoritarian style than hitherto would be implemented. This would depend very much on the extent to which Health Authorities chose to recognize the need to encourage the principle of General Managers working through managers who specialized in single fields of activity.

Within the new general management system, RHA and DHA Chairmen were to be given greater freedom to organize the management structure of the Health Authorities in the way best suited to local requirements and management potential. Units would play key roles in the decision-making process, which would be brought closer to the locality for which services were being provided. Each Unit of Management would have a total budget and would develop management budgets involving doctors, and relate workload and service objectives to financial and manpower allocations.

Although General Managers were to be appointed at Regional and District level, it was the Unit general management function which would be the source of a dilemma concerning the organization and management of physiotherapy services.

Physiotherapy management

In Districts where there was a District Physiotherapy Manager, service was provided, managed and co-ordinated across Unit and specialty boundaries. Post-holders were generally responsible for managing the District physiotherapy budget, personnel, equipment and facilities; budgetary resources, staff and equipment could usually be moved across Unit boundaries. In some Health Authorities, a Designated District Physiotherapist was appointed to advise District management teams on physiotherapy matters; such designates had no managerial responsibility, as confirmed by DS 331/75, *Designation of Therapists* (DHSS 1975).[14] In some Health Authorities, there were no District or Designated District Physiotherapists; in these authorities, management of physiotherapy services happened on a piecemeal and fragmented basis (*see* Chapter 1).

The District Physiotherapist was the professional leader, both managerially and clinically. He/she was responsible for input into the District planning cycle, implementation of DHSS, RHA and DHA policies, making sure that the physiotherapy function was geared into the overall objectives of the organization and for a wide range of managerial, administrative and consultancy duties. Figure 4.3 shows a typical Health Authority management structure, including the position of the District Physiotherapist relative to other managers (pre-Griffiths). Clinical leadership and management were important aspects of the District Physiotherapist's role. Postholders were clinical heads of clinical services, the leaders and professional directors whose major concerns were for patient care. The day-to-day work of the District Physiotherapist consisted largely of actions and decisions about patients and clinical matters, there being an inextricable link between these clinical and managerial roles.

General management and physiotherapy management

Under the Griffiths proposals, the Units of mangement were to be the focus for the impact of general management. UGMs were to be accountable for drawing together planning, implementation and control of performance, and would have overall responsibility for the total unit budget. One objective of Unit management was to bring decision-making closer to the patients than had been the case under DMTs. The view of the Chartered Society of Physiotherapy was that to be clinically effective it was necessary for physiotherapy services to be managed on a District-wide basis. However, under the Griffiths initiatives, Health Authorities would institute management structures based at the Unit rather than District level.

Before the advent of Griffiths, the majority of DHAs had chosen to employ a District Physiotherapist (*see* Chapter 1). With the move towards basing management structures at Unit rather than District level, a question would arise about the level at which physiotherapy services should be managed, 'for some activities, it would clearly be widely uneconomic to have each Unit with its own department. Also it seems that some functions . . . need a District presence so that uniformity of policy and practice can be ensured' (Dixon 1983).[15]

As well as the important factors concerning the economics of managing physiotherapy and uniformity of service provision across all Units within a District, there would be many other matters of concern to physiotherapists and General Managers alike.

When the Griffiths Report was published, District Physiotherapists had been undertaking most of these duties and responsibilities and had been doing so for some years.

The philosophy of general management meant that decisions would be made as near to the patient as possible and, in order to achieve this, the major focus for decision-making was to be at Unit rather than District level. The UGM

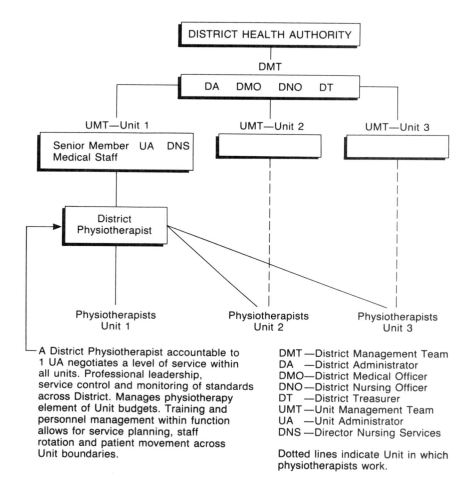

Figure 4.3. The District Physiotherapist relative to the District Management Structure—pre Griffiths

would be accountable for the overall planning, service provision and performance of the Unit. It might, therefore, be argued that UGMs would need full managerial control over the PAMs. However, it was the type and level of this control, the managerial relationship between them and the proposed organizational structures, that raised questions for General Managers and physiotherapists alike.

Questions such as:

Who would manage the physiotherapy budget?

Who would be responsible and accountable for the effectiveness and efficiency of physiotherapy services and ensure the quality of service provision?

What would be the mechanism for physiotherapy service accountability to the DHA?

How would physiotherapy services be monitored and who would be responsible for this?

What would be the mechanism for the development and planning of physiotherapy services and the implementation of new initiatives?

Who would be responsible for the implementation of DHSS, RHA and DHA initiatives and policies such as Körner, Patient Audit and Problem Orientated Medical Records?

Who would be responsible for managing clinical supervision of physiotherapy students and liaise with training schools?

Who would undertake physiotherapy staff personnel work including staff recruitment interviewing, writing job descriptions, etc.?

How would physiotherapy research projects be set up and managed?

Who would advise on and manage physiotherapy staff training?

What would be the mechanism for dealing with complaints about physiotherapy services?

Who would be responsible for physiotherapy staff development and appraisal—Individual Performance Review (IPR)?

Who would be responsible for ensuring the most economical use of resources; personnel—including staff deployment—equipment and facilities?

Who would be responsible for physiotherapy marketing?

Who would be responsible for initiating and managing the physiotherapy information system?

5 The National Health Service and Community Care Act 1990. An Overview
S.A. Philbrook

The National Health Service (NHS) and Community Care Bill, which encompasses the most radical shake up of the NHS since its inception, received the Royal Assent on 29 June 1990 with most of the legislation due to take effect from April 1991.

The bill was based on three White Papers. *Working for Patients* (DoH 1989)[1] and *Caring for People* (DoH 1989)[2] were published during 1989 and deal with the reform of health and social care in hospital and the community. These papers were preceded by the publication in 1987 of *Promoting Better Health* (DHSS 1987)[3] which proposed changes to Family Practitioner Committees—now called Family Health Services Authorities (FHSAs)—services and care that general practitioners (GPs), dentists, opticians and pharmacists deliver in the context of primary health care. Together, these papers are set to change all aspects of the way in which care is provided in the UK.

The philosophy which underlies the changes is that the consumer will be given greater choice and increased involvement in the services provided.

A review of the health service was announced by the Prime Minister in 1988 following mounting pressure concerning the funding of the service. *Working for Patients* was, therefore, born out of the need to review funding, but it has not addressed this issue. Instead it has sought, by changing the funding arrangements—which will now be based on a weighted per capita basis in which money will follow the patient and the introduction of an internal market—to introduce competition into health care. The White Paper has been followed by a series of working papers which seek to give more detail to the original proposals.

The long-awaited *Caring for People* White Paper was published some 18 months after Sir Roy Griffiths' Report *Community Care Agenda for Action* (DHSS 1988)[4] and formed the Government's response to the report's proposals. The original spur to this report had been the findings of the Audit Commission of inefficiency and misdirection in the current system of funding of residential care through social security.

To implement the reforms, Health and Local Authorities are to take on commissioning or purchasing roles. They will determine what local services are needed and decide on what services to buy to meet that need for their population. Joint planning between both authorities will now take on a much more strategic and vital role, and plans will have to be complementary. It will be crucial to foster collaborative working arrangements within the operational or provider services, particularly in the difficult divide between health and social care. Commissioning/Purchasing Authorities will be at arms length from the providers of care.

The purchasers—Commissioning Authorities

Regional and District Health Authorities

The current role of RHAs and DHAs is largely undefined. In future, the size of authorities will be reduced and they will retain a chairman appointed by the Secretary of State. Management of services will be less directed from the centre with Health Authorities taking on this role and the responsibility for implementing the changes. At the centre, the management executive has set the agenda and in this way *Working for Patients* is intrinsically different from previous White Papers. Formerly, objectives were set and included a detailed prescription as to how they were to be achieved, but now local managers are left to exploit policy by local initiative. This method of change is common in the commercial sector, but has not been used before in this country in public health care.

The diminished membership of Health Authorities will consist of executive members, to include the General Manager and the Finance Director, and non-executive members appointed on the basis of the experience they can bring to the running of a complex organization. The local community will continue to be represented by Community Health Councils; however, the Local Authority does not retain membership.

In an executive letter of March 1989 Duncan Nicol, as Chief Executive of the Health Service, identified five key areas for DHAs to ensure:

- that the health needs of their population are met;
- that there are effective services for the prevention and control of disease and the promotion of health;
- that their population has access to a comprehensive range of high-quality, value-for-money services;
- that targets are set and performance against them monitored in those Units for which they continue to have responsibility;
- that an effective system of medical audit is in place and undertaking responsibility for the day-to-day management of their consultants' contracts.

Family Practitioner Committees—Family Health Services Authorities

Prior to these changes Family Practitioner Committees (FPCs) have acted primarily as pay bodies playing a limited part in the planning and monitoring of primary health care. Accountability for these services—now lying with the Department of Health—will move to regions, along with the introduction of general management in to FHSAs.

The Act and the new contracts for practitioners alter substantially the role and tasks of the FHSA and the environment in which services are provided. They are now required to identify, along with Health Authorities, the health needs of the local population and use resources actively to support practitioners with the aim of high-quality responsive care. The contracts contain a requirement to achieve targets for health promotional activity, particularly in respect of the screening of children and elderly people, which are linked to financial rewards.

GPs with lists of more than 11,000 patients are free to apply for NHS budgets in order to obtain a specified range of services from the NHS or private sector; these include, out-patients, a defined group of in- and day-patient care services, and some diagnostic tests. Additionally, there will be changes in the funding of practice staff, giving an opportunity to employ a range of professionals, budgets for drugs, and the cost rent scheme for the improvement of practice premises.

Local Authorities

Social Services, together with Health Authorities and FHSAs, are asked to ensure that 'seamless' services are available to people in their care. The extent of these arrangements should allow choice and effective targeting of resources. Taking the lead in the arrangements for social care does not mean that Social Services have to provide the care.

The Community Care Report *Agenda for Action* (DHSS 1988)[5] proposed that the provision of care at the public's expense should be preceded by proper assessment of individual needs. Sir Roy Griffiths' vision was that the authorities should be the arrangers and purchasers of care rather than monopolistic providers. By working with a range of providers in the statutory (not for profit) and private sectors they would act as enablers, developing their purchasing and contracting role.

Case management is at the centre of care in the community and the Government's view is that it will provide an effective method for directing resources and planning services to meet the specific individual requirements of a client. Case management encompasses a holistic assessment of need—physical, social and psychological—involving the views of the individuals themselves and carers. Case management is a continuous process made up of an initial assessment, monitoring and reassessment adapting to changing need. Flexibility is, therefore, essential.

The providers

In this new approach, the operational services are to become the provider services. Managers of health care will move away from delivery within the policies and budget of a particular authority to delivery contracted services, within quantity and quality specifications, to one or a number of clients in return for agreed levels of income.

Within this framework of increasingly delegated responsibility and the role of the provider, services have the opportunity to become self-governing outside Health Authority control, but still within the NHS. Such units, to be called Trusts, will be governed by Boards of Directors and have greater flexibility in the services offered, who they employ and over the terms and conditions of those that they employ. Revenue will be generated by income from services provided to a range of clients—GPs, the public and private sector. Units which do not take on self-government will remain under Health Authority direction and be given the epithet Directly Managed Unit (DMU).

Accompanying the ability for self-government, and to bring the NHS more into line with the commercial sector, proposals for the charging of capital assets have been introduced. This is seen as a way of facilitating competition between sectors and for the NHS to use its capital more effectively. Capital charges have two components:

1 depreciation on assets;
2 interest calculated on the current value of the capital assets used by authorities.

Consequently, during the early part of 1990 capital asset registers of all buildings and equipment within the NHS have been drawn up and will act as a base for initial costings.

Contracts

The basis for the management of the service will be the contract between the purchaser and the provider. The purchasers will specify the services they wish to buy for their resident population. Each provider organization—hospital, Unit, function—will produce a specification which describes what they will supply to the purchaser. The contract will seek to guarantee:

● the appropriateness of the care;
● the effectiveness of the service;

- the timeliness of the provision;
- the accessibility to the customer;
- the continuity of care through assessment, diagnosis, intervention and aftercare;
- the acceptability of the service to the customer.

Any contract will contain a cost, including both capital and revenue costs, quantity and quality components. In drawing up service specifications, managers will have to include an analysis of possible local competitors and/or alternative ways of delivering services; develop standards, outcome and quality measures and quality assurance programmes in order to safeguard consumers' interests.

Purchasers come from a wide range of sources. There is the obvious patient/client relationship, but also clinicians and GPs as customers of other types of services, both clinical and general.

The divide between purchasers and providers has brought into focus the way in which many services are currently provided. Not least of these are all aspects of education and training. Education and training will also be governed by contracts. Pre-registration education contracts may be set on the outcome of the numbers of successful students, but must also include professional and academic criteria if quality is to be ensured. Contracts for clinical placements will be held between colleges and services. Post-registration education, in many cases a covert uncosted process, will need to become a costed overt process with measurable outcomes.

Manpower planning for 'key' professional and technical staff has been set on the basis of regional self-sufficiency. Contracts set in this way will need to take into account the mobility of staff with greater opportunity to be employed outside the public sector.

Medical audit

Within *Working for Patients*, there is a commitment to medical audit. Described as a systematic critical analysis of the quality of medical care widened to include all the other professions, it will allow the steady drive to implement standards, the recognition of high-quality services and improvements in others. The legislation allows the setting up of a national clinical standards group with membership drawn only from the Royal Colleges and advisory councils.

Resources

The Government's stated intention is to retain services as largely tax financed and with health care mostly free at the point of use. Funding arrangements for social care are to change with Local Authorities responsible for managing a single unified budget, basing use on assessment. Individuals may be able to claim support from Income Support and Housing Benefit.

From 1991, the audit arrangements for Health Authorities and FHSAs will be transferred to an independent body, the Audit Commission, which is currently responsible for the audit of Local Authorities in England and Wales. The plan to transfer audit from the DoH is a further push by the Government to achieve better value for money.

Great stock is placed on the use of staff and the provision of appropriate education and training at all levels. Working in collaboration with the National Council for Vocational Qualifications, established by the Government in 1986, Health and Social Services are members of the Care Sector consortium which is intending to secure a recognized pattern of qualification for all those working in community care. Many new staff will be required to support the contracting processes—business planners, accountants and information specialists.

In looking for value for money, *Working for Patients* is clear that those people who make decisions should be accountable for their spending, that those who manage services should be able to influence how resources are used and that decisions are best made at a local level.

Resource management

The introduction of general management promoted the concept of management budgeting, costing by speciality and the setting up of a number of pilot sites for its implementation. Within the pilot Districts, there was a move away from functional budgeting to budget holding by individual doctors who took responsibility for expenditure. This process encountered many problems and in 1986 the Resource Management Initiative (RMI) was launched (*see* Chapter 7).

Audit primarily by peer review is part and parcel of resource management and should flow from project implementation. It is given a further stimulus in the White Papers directing that each Health Authority and FHSA set up a committee for audit by April 1991. The outcomes of audit can make significant changes both in practice and to the use of resources. There is obviously a place for single-discipline audit, but if audit is widened to all other professions involved in health care, great advances in collaboration and patient care could be made.

Information

Underpinning all these reforms is the need for more and more relevant information. Implementation of the proposals will require support by appropriate information derived from objectives, functions and processes. The central feature—the contracting operation—will require information based on the resident population as well as the patient/client population. Data will be necessary in respect of patient/client cross-boundary flows, the financial implication of a decision and the ability to compare outcomes. Some national uniformity is, therefore, necessary. Providers will require data to assist contract planning, formulation and the monitoring of procedures.

Systems will be necessary to aid the management of a wide range of activities that have been generated by the two White Papers, for example, screening, capital asset registers, identification of the payer, clinical audit and for GPs who become fund holders.

With the implementation of this Act, the Government is seeking a major cultural shift in a very short space of time. There will be a move to a business enterprise commercial ethos in order to provide consumer orientated high-quality services—a free market philosophy based on value for money and choice. The theme running through the White Papers is choice. However, actual consumer alternatives will be governed by the purchasing agencies who are set to act on the public's behalf. Only time will tell if these reforms will succeed and the major upheaval that the services are experiencing will actually give the public the facility of option and variety of choice.

6 Legal Aspects in Physiotherapy
A.P. Andrews

Legal aspects

Law, these days, has a very high profile and scarcely a day passes without some reference to the law or legal process in the media. There is little doubt that society is becoming increasingly litigious and patients are becoming increasingly aware of their rights. It is against this background that physiotherapists ask the question, 'Where do I stand in all this?' Most claims against Health Authorities and their staff allege negligence and in this chapter we shall be looking at the general principles which underlie the concepts of negligence and of the duty of care.

Negligence can be quite simply defined as an act or an omission from which there follows foreseeable harm. It is important to remember that negligence can be just as much the doing as the failure to do. This can be quite simply illustrated by two recent cases. A nurse working in the community visited a mother and baby; she decided the baby's mouth needed cleaning, took some cotton wool, placed it on the end of a pair of scissors and proceeded, with the result that the child suffered irrevocable palate damage. This clearly is an illustration of negligence by act. Contrast that with the case of a physiotherapist to whom a patient was referred for ultraviolet light treatment. Three minutes exposure had been prescribed by the physiotherapist, prone and supine. The first three minutes were given; the patient, who was extremely drowsy, was then turned and the physiotherapist decided that she had time to make a quick telephone call. She took a timer with her and was on the telephone for no more than 70 seconds. However, on her way back to the patient she was waylaid by a colleague, became involved in other activities in the department and to her horror remembered the patient some 30 minutes later. Here, we have an illustration of negligence by omission.

For the purposes of the law, the test of foreseeability is always an objective and not a subjective one. All too often staff will say, 'but I meant well' or 'I acted in good faith'. In seeking to establish the foreseeability, one does not look at the intention, but rather applies the test of the official bystander with knowledge; in other words, what would someone looking on have reasonably foreseen? There can be no doubt that in the two examples we have looked at the health professionals intended no harm to their respective patients. Nevertheless, anybody standing back and analysing the situation could have anticipated what ultimately happened and, therefore, from a legal point of view it would have been foreseeable.

In essence, the law of negligence is based on the good neighbour principle, which says that an individual owes a duty of care to his neighbour. The term 'neighbour' is construed almost in a biblical sense in that anybody who is affected by your acts or omissions is, in law, your neighbour and owed a duty of care. In the context of your work, this means that you owe a duty of care to each and every patient in your charge. If asked to define precisely what constitutes this duty of care, a simple answer might be to say that you owe the duty of care which would be shown by a reasonable man or a reasonable woman, and in the context of a profession an individual will be judged against someone with his knowledge, experience and qualifications. If there is a question about precisely what constitutes the duty of care, ultimately it is the profession which determines that issue. When a case comes to court the plaintiff (the person suing) will seek to find the most eminent members of the profession who will say, 'but no right thinking physiotherapist would have acted in that way' and if you are to defend the action successfully you will need equally eminent experts who will say 'This is precisely what I would have expected from a physiotherapist given the situation.' In other words, the acid test when tempted to do something untoward must always be to ask, 'Can I justify my actions now to my professional colleagues?' If the answer to that question is no, the professional is immediately vulnerable, but if he knows that the profession would endorse what he has decided to do, he should have little anxiety about being able to justify the course of action he has embarked upon.

It is a characteristic of the professional that he or she cannot plead superior orders. In other words, one cannot escape liability by saying, 'But I was only doing what my boss told me to do' or 'This is what I was instructed to do by the doctor.' If a professional embarks on any treatment, his only justification for doing so is that he is professionally satisfied that it is both right and appropriate. In the field of health care, there is always considerable difficulty as a result of working alongside many other disciplines, and it is important to be quite clear in your own mind about the extent of your professional responsibilities.

The National Health Service (NHS) Act 1977 imposes a duty on the Secretary of State to provide a comprehensive and integrated Health Service and he delegates these functions through RHAs to Districts and it is, therefore, the DHA which owes its patients a duty of care. Clearly, the Authority itself cannot provide that care on a day-to-day basis and entrusts the responsibility for that to its professional staff, who are, in effect, the hands, eyes and ears of the Authority. Thus, although it is very tempting for a professional to claim ownership of a patient, it is important to remember that the patient is ultimately the responsibility of the Health Authority, who will continue to owe a duty of care regardless of what particular member of staff may be in a post at any time.

In the multidisciplinary setting, therefore, it is important to define precisely the sphere of responsibility of each professional. Within his respective sphere, he must be supreme. While others can urge, counsel or persuade, they cannot direct, because responsibility and accountability rests with the individual practitioner. For a physiotherapist, this will mean that he or she will receive a referral from a doctor which will specify a medical diagnosis (*see* Chapter 3), which is entirely the responsibility of the doctor, and a request for treatment as appropriate. If a doctor purports to order a particular treatment, this does not constitute an instruction to the physiotherapist, but must be regarded as a recommendation. If the physiotherapist is unhappy or not prepared to carry out such treatment, it is encumbent on her to go back to the referrer and say that she will not be proceeding, giving reasons for that decision. It must be remembered that, whilst the doctor cannot direct the treatment that will be given, because he has overall responsibility for the well-being of the patient, it is open to him to withdraw the referral if he is so minded.

The word 'accountability' is very much in vogue at present and perhaps, therefore, has become overused. What in essence is meant is that a professional is individually answerable for what he or she has done or chosen not to do and his/her acts or omissions will ultimately be weighed in the balance, and when they are so weighed, the question to be asked is, 'Will the professional be found wanting?' Essentially, when seeking to establish whether or not negligence has occurred the question will be asked, 'Has the individual met the required professional standard or fallen short of that?'

There is a common expectation on the part of the public that whenever something goes wrong there will be an automatic entitlement to compensation as a result of the wrong done. In reality this is not so. Fundamental to the concept of negligence is the notion of fault. An error of judgment does not constitute negligence. We hope as a result of the intervention of health professionals that patients will benefit. Some sadly will not because ultimately care involves risk taking. There are many situations which occur on almost a daily basis to illustrate that point. Today, for the first time, it is decided that a patient will walk unaided, with disastrous results. As part of rehabilitation, a patient is sent out into the community unsupervised, only to be knocked down by a car. A psychiatric patient is discharged and within two hours he commits suicide. The list is endless. But while all of these will quite properly be matters of regret, they are not necessarily matters of fault. That will be determined not by the outcome, but by looking at the decision-making process that led up to the ultimate event.

A further characteristic of the professional is the ability to recognize the limits of his or her competence and to have the courage to say 'no' when lacking expertise or practical experience to deal with the situation with which confronted. At the same time, a professional is required to keep up to date and abreast of developments in his own field, and judges have often said, 'Conduct will be judged in the light of knowledge which was then—or ought to have been—possessed' and just as experts will tell the court what constitutes good professional practice, so these same experts will also be used to talk about the state of knowledge at the time of the alleged wrong. In this context it should, however, be remembered that the important question to be addressed is, 'What was the state of knowledge at the time of the alleged wrong?' It is not permissible to judge yesterday's activities by today's standards.

Although, in theory, an action for negligence could be directed at the individual professional who is alleged to have done wrong, in practice this seldom if ever happens, the plaintiff relying on the doctrine of vicarious liability. What this means is that when an individual acts in a representative capacity his or her principal is legally liable for his wrongful acts or omissions. In the context of employment, this means that an employer is liable for the acts and omissions of his employees and, therefore, provided the professional was acting within the scope of his employment, he can look to his employer to indemnify him against any claims arising from the care or treatment he has given. If an employee is negligent in the performance of his duties, his employer is nevertheless still liable, because the law takes the view that he has not been adequately supervised.

Although the law allows an employer to exercise a right of relief against an employee who has done wrong, enabling him, therefore, to recover from him any damages he may have had to pay out, the Secretary of State has made it clear that this course of action will not be pursued by Health Authorities. If, however, an employee without the knowledge of his employer undertakes activities which it is no part of his work to do, the law will regard him as having embarked upon an enterprise of his own and he cannot, in those circumstances, look to his employer for indemnity.

Once a patient has been accepted by the physiotherapist for treatment, the duty owed to that individual by the professional is absolute and it would be no defence for the physiotherapist to say he did not give appropriate care due to lack of facilities or lack of resources. This means that the physiotherapist will need to assess the likely demands which the patient is anticipated to make and to ensure that he does not accept so many patients for treatment that he does not give them the care which he knows professionally they need. Any decision as to treatment must be based on professional grounds and not on expediency. There is no legal requirement that the NHS responds to every identified need on demand. What is required is that a reasonable provision is made within the resources available to the Health Authority and when resources are limited it is the responsibility of managers to identify and set priorities.

One of the problems facing staff who are involved in litigation is that the claim may often be brought many years after the events to which it relates.

A civil action is determined by a judge on the balance of probabilities, in other words, he has got to say ultimately, 'Who has got the best evidence and whom do I believe?' Faced with a plaintiff who on oath remembers everything and a physiotherapist who remembers little or nothing about the events, the plaintiff will inevitably win. The answer to this problem lies in the physiotherapist's notes and professionals need to remember that everything which they write in the course of their work has the potential status of a legal document and may at some time see the light of day in a court. If an action is brought, the notes will be scrutinized long before witnesses are seen and, depending on the nature of the notes, some initial views will inevitably be formed. If notes or records are found to be less than professional, it is almost inevitable that someone will seek to suggest that a similar failure applies to the care and treatment which was given to the patient. The purpose of the record is to facilitate the care, treatment and support of the patient. No one health professional has total responsibility for the well-being of the patient. This is a shared responsibility and the records which are an integral part of care are the means by which efficient communication takes place. Ideally, one physiotherapist's record will show precisely where she is with an individual patient. She will then play her part, which must be recorded, and other physiotherapists coming after her will likewise be able to follow on. Staff are often worried about the significance of their entries and seem unsure what ought to be recorded. Bearing in mind the purpose of the record, the practical answer must be to ask the question, 'If I were coming to this patient without any knowledge for the first time what would I need to know?' If the information satisfies this criterion, it must be included in the record. If it is incidental to that, it is not worthy of note. The notes need to record both achievements and failures, and even where care is proceeding on a continuous basis and following an agreed plan the note will need to indicate that this has taken place and who is responsible on this occasion. It is important that entries are authenticated so that practitioners can be clearly identified at a later date. Occasionally, records are compiled merely with a series of ticks or crosses, without any indication of who has made the entry or indeed when that occurred, and from an evidential point of view this is of no value whatever.

Professionals in a managed service often face a conflict between instructions which they receive from management and the discharge of their professional duty of care. It must be management's prerogative to state what must be done; however, it is entirely a matter for a professional to decide how it is to be achieved and no manager can direct an individual as to the discharge of his professional responsibilities. While it is good practice to follow laid down policies and procedures, and one would expect a good physiotherapist to do so, these must never be followed blindly. To respond in such a way would, in effect, be pleading superior orders and if professional practice amounts to no more than following policies and procedures one questions whether training would be necessary at all! No policy or procedure can ever deal with every eventuality and the physiotherapist needs to be alert to the fact that the day will surely dawn when, for whatever reason, she will recognize that the established procedure is manifestly inappropriate. What is important is that when she decides to depart from laid down policies and procedures she is satisfied that there is professional justification for that decision and it has not been done merely as a matter of expediency. Thus, in seeking to explain her actions, while it would be inappropriate to hide behind policies and procedures, there is no doubt that they can be used as a very strong reinforcement when she says, 'I formed a professional view, and what is more, this is endorsed by policies and procedures'.

Although physiotherapists may now receive referrals from a variety of sources including self-referral and referral from other health care professions and carers – in the context of their employment they must comply with their Health Authority's instructions; sometimes such instructions may be more prescriptive than those permitted by the professional body. There are some authorities which restrict referrals, either to medical staff or to medical staff and other disciplines. In other areas, there operates what is sometimes referred to as 'blanket referrals', where the physiotherapist has access to any patient as of right and will make his own judgment as to whether any intervention is required. From a professional point of view, this latter system does carry certain risks for the physiotherapist if the number of potential patients is so great that he cannot adequately monitor what is happening to them all.

While it is the professional's responsibility to determine what treatment ought to be given, he cannot proceed without the consent of the patient. For consent to be effective, the physiotherapist needs to be satisfied that the patient understands the nature, purpose and likely outcome of the proposed treatment. There is no legal requirement that consent be given in any particular form and, indeed, many situations will routinely occur where consent is given by implication or by word of mouth. The value of a written consent is purely evidential in that if there is a signed consent in the notes this will speak for itself and there will be no other need to prove consent in any other way. As a matter of law, no adult can consent on behalf of another and once an individual has reached the age of 18 chronologically, regardless of mental ability, the law regards that person to be an adult. In an emergency, where it is necessary to intervene to preserve life or limb, there is no difficulty, since the defence of necessity will apply to that situation and no formal consent will be required.

The real problem arises when dealing with an adult who, for whatever reason, is incapable of giving consent and treatment is not immediately necessary to deal with an emergency. As a matter of good practice, it is sensible to go to the next of kin, simply because if a patient is incapable of giving consent in all probability he will also be incapable of suing. Any action on the patient's behalf would be brought by the next of kin in a representative capacity and if the next of kin is party to the decision to treat, it is unlikely they will wish to sue. In those cases where there is no relative, the health professional, before proceeding to treat without consent in the non-urgent situation, should always obtain a second opinion from a fellow professional not directly involved with the care of that patient in order to confirm that the proposed treatment is in the patient's best interest. In the case of minors (up to the age of 18 years), consent will be given by the parent or guardian, but the Family Law Reform Act provides that a child who has attained his or her 16th birthday can give effective consent to surgical, medical or dental treatment. This provision, however, does not affect the legal position of the parent or guardian and the effect is that from birth to 16 years, consent will come from parent or guardian, while from 18 years of age on, it will come from the patient only. In the two-year period of 16–18 years two consents are possible, either the parent or guardian or the patient. The problem of conflict has not been addressed by Parliament, but it should be remembered that consent is an authority to proceed and not a veto and, therefore, provided a consent comes from either party, the treatment would be lawful and the only practical advice one can give staff in that situation is to act in the best interest of the patient.

Some questions answered

1. What is the legal position concerning physiotherapists responding to letters from solicitors?

As a general rule, physiotherapists who are in employment should not answer letters from solicitors on an individual personal basis on matters relating to their work. Most authorities will have an established procedure whereby all requests for information from solicitors are channelled through a nominated individual, who will consider the request and respond appropriately. Any request for information must be accompanied by the patient's authority to disclose the information sought and in reaching a decision on whether or not to provide the information or report, the physiotherapist will need to know for what purpose the information is required. Often, information is needed by the patient for the purposes of pursuing a claim against a third party and in such situations authorities are expected to co-operate fully. If, however, the information is needed in connection with an action or proposed action against the employing Authority, advice should be sought from the Authority's legal advisers before any response is made. Should a decision be made not to co-operate, it is unlikely that the physiotherapist will be involved in subsequent proceedings, since lawyers are generally reluctant to subpoena a witness unless they have some clear indication of the evidence that he or she is likely to give. Once an opinion has been put to paper, even if the physiotherapist then gets cold feet and decides not to assist further, it will be too late. The solicitor will know the tenor of the information, have some indication of her views and can compel attendance at court by means of subpoena or witness summons if he thinks it would be helpful to his client's cause. The provision of advice and information of this kind does not form part of the service which Authorities are required to provide under the NHS Acts and it is for that reason that discretion exists in dealing with requests of this nature.

2. **What are the legal implications of the physiotherapist's report as part of the 'statementing' process for children under the Education Act 1981, and what are the physiotherapist's legal responsibilities under this Act?**

By virtue of the Education Act 1981, physiotherapists, along with other health professionals, are required to submit a report identifying a child's needs. This must be an objective professional assessment and must not be influenced in any way by the known facilities and resources which would be available to treat the child. The report should be regarded as setting out the ideal treatment which the physiotherapist considers would provide optimum benefit to the child. Although it is a statutory requirement to identify the child's needs, the Health Authority, unlike the Education Authority, is not obliged to meet that need once identified. The requirement imposed on the Authority by the statute is to meet the child's needs within the resources available to it. It follows, therefore, that in some cases a child might receive either less treatment than the ideal or indeed none at all. The matter is further complicated by the fact that the original statement is a matter of professional judgment and if, subsequently, a child is accepted for treatment, the receiving physiotherapist will make her own assessment as to the treatment which should be given and this need not coincide with the need originally identified.

3. **What is the legal position concerning fees for reports on patients when it is agreed that a physiotherapist's report will be submitted to a solicitor?**

If a report is submitted to a solicitor because it falls outside the scope of services which an Authority is required to give, a fee may be charged. Given that the report will in all probability be prepared in the employer's time and that it relates to matters arising directly out of the physiotherapist's employment, any fees for reports on individual patients who have been treated are the Authority's. If, on the other hand, a physiotherapist is acting as an expert witness and giving a professional view on a case with which she has not been involved, provided this is done in her own time, the fee which is negotiated with the solicitor will be hers to keep.

4. What are the legal implications involved in physiotherapists' teaching activities in, for example, lifting training, ergonomic advice, to other working groups within the NHS and outside it?

When a physiotherapist undertakes activities of this nature, either because it is a requirement imposed on her by her employer or because it is an activity which she undertakes on a private basis in her own time, the physiotherapist, by undertaking the task, warrants that she has the skill, qualifications and expertise necessary to do so. In other words, the training must be of an appropriate professional standard which will stand scrutiny by her peers. If, as a result of such training, an individual claiming to have acted as taught then comes to grief, he will need to establish fault if he is to have any prospect of success in claiming damages from the physiotherapist. Should the matter proceed to court, the judge will determine the issue on the balance of probabilities. In other words, he will have to weigh up who has the best evidence and whom, ultimately, he believes. Invariably, the plaintiff has a very clear recollection of everything which occurred during the session, while the physiotherapist will be unable to recall the session in any detail. Very often, the plaintiff's account of what occurred is not truly accurate. No sinister motive is imputed to this. The memory is frail and, with time, it is a perfectly natural tendency to rationalize events which occurred in the past and, ultimately, to believe that modified or edited account. It is, therefore, of the utmost importance that physiotherapists who undertake such teaching maintain full and accurate records detailing exactly what was taught and what practical instruction and guidance was given, because faced with a professional with good records, it would be hard to overcome the presumption that, in the event of conflicting accounts, the professional's is the version to be preferred.

Despite the most careful training, the process of lifting is still attended with risk and many groups of staff who are required to carry out this activity, in the normal course of their duties, may well experience back injury at some stage. Indeed, one might well regard it as an occupational hazard for some professions within the NHS. It is a well-established legal principle that if somebody knowingly and voluntarily accepts a risk and then the worst happens, they have no legal redress. Clearly, any accident involving a member of staff must be a matter of regret and injuries sustained in the course of work are the subject of specific provisions in the Whitley Agreements, which are over and above any statutory benefits to which the employee may be entitled as a result of his/her disability. To obtain further compensation through the courts, that individual would need to establish a breach of the duty of care owed to him by the trainer.

7 Information Systems and Resource Management
R.J. Jones

Information systems and resource management are very complex subjects. Each could easily be a book in its own right. There are many possible approaches to the development of systems in physiotherapy; it is the purpose of this chapter to focus on the most important aspects and to provide guidelines on some of the issues to be considered. This is not a prescription, nor is it claimed that the approach outlined is the only way forward.

Introduction to information systems in physiotherapy

The primary function of physiotherapy is the provision of a clinical service. However, over the past few years information systems have become increasingly important in the NHS and consequently also in physiotherapy. For nearly 40 years, statistics about physiotherapy activity were collected on Form SH3 which asked for figures on new patients and 'attendances' by in- and out-patients only.

The impetus for the development of information systems in physiotherapy was provided by the NHS/DHSS Steering Group on Health Services Information which was chaired by Mrs Edith Körner and reported during the period 1983–1985. The data collection requirements laid down in the Körner reports for England and Wales gave rise to the development of a variety of paper-based and computerized systems for capturing and processing this information. Some systems have been designed by physiotherapists to suit national requirements and local needs, while others are the result of modifications to existing systems used by other disciplines and adapted for physiotherapy use. Two things are certain: firstly, that Physiotherapy Managers will be required to establish systems capable of collecting a wide variety of information and, secondly, that there is no 'right' or 'only one' way of doing it.

Main factors for consideration in physiotherapy information systems design

Chartered Physiotherapists employed in the NHS work in a wide variety of health care settings, and the scope and spectrum of modern practice is both diverse and complex. For these and other reasons, the process of data recording, collection, sorting, collation, reporting, interpreting and storage is also likely to be complex and involved. There are many factors which must be weighed when designing efficient and relevant physiotherapy computerized information systems. Some of the main aspects for consideration are listed below.

- The systems must be 'owned' by the physiotherapists using them locally and be developed in accordance with physiotherapy clinical and managerial practices.
- All information collected must be for identified use—decide what you really need and want.
- The system needs to provide the information required nationally, regionally and locally, by the DoH, RHA, DHA (commissioning or purchasing authority) and Units (service providers).
- Systems must be computerized in order to cope with the volume and diversity of data, and the computer must be large enough to cope with the volume of work and variety of uses.
- Systems must be capable of processing information relevant to the management of physiotherapy services and clinical practice.
- The data capture paperwork must be uncomplicated and user friendly.
- The paperwork system for clinical use and data capture must be uniform across as large a locality as possible—the same paperwork to be used in hospitals, community, schools and every other site is most efficient.
- The information collected must be, as far as possible, the by-product of clinical activity so that the minimum of clinical time is lost through data collection.
- For quality assurance; to facilitate clinical audit and research including recording and analysis of outcome measures (see Chapter 9).
- To encompass the Problem Orientated Medical Records (POMR) system (see Chapter 9).
- To interface with RMI projects.
- To facilitate the development of costing and pricing mechanisms in accordance with physiotherapy practice.
- To maintain strong links with the companies writing software for physiotherapy systems to ensure relevant and desirable development.
- To ensure that systems are capable of incorporating the most up-to-date approaches to physiotherapy clinical and managerial practice.
- Computer systems must have the capacity for modules which will permit, for example, electronic mail, word processing, spreadsheets and graphics.
- There must be capacity to include management modules for physiotherapy personnel management, travel (mileages), training, leavers, joiners and so on.

- It is helpful to be aware of recent developments in technology when considering system design and application so that new developments can be incorporated when necessary or when they can be afforded. One example of this is Optical Character Recognition (OCR) which may eventually take over the reading of completed data slips into the computer rather than the information being keyed in by a clerical officer.

Körner requirements

The Körner NHS/DHSS Steering Group produced six reports and three supplementary reports on Health Services information. The main reports were:

- Hospital Clinical Services (K1);
- Patient Transport Services (K2);
- Manpower Information (K3);
- Paramedical Services and Other Issues (K4);
- Community Health Services (K5);
- Finance Information (K6).

The reports most relevant to physiotherapy were K3, K4 and K6. Three main types of statistical information about physiotherapy were identified:

1 data about physiotherapy manpower (K3 and K4);
2 data about what the physiotherapists do and the patients they treat (activity statistics) (K4);
3 data about 'what it costs' (financial information) (K6).

Körner (3 and 4) proposed the collection of data for manpower purposes on, for example, absence from work and reasons for leaving. This sort of information is generally collected direct by employing authorities through the time sheet, termination and appointment form mechanisms, for which Physiotherapy Managers are responsible. This information is not generally processed by 'dedicated' physiotherapy computer systems, but rather by the manpower and finance computers in Health Authority or Unit Headquarters. Figure 7.1 overleaf is an example of a summary report of staff absences during one month.

Physiotherapy staff activity—the sample inquiry

One of the requirements for the PAMs laid down in the Fourth Körner Report is the collection of information about staff activity; this is to be carried out at least once a year for a sample period.

Total Physiotherapy   Month End: April 1990

Post/ Grade	WTE Staff in Post	Sickness			Sickness Per cent Absent	Leave and Training							Leave/ Training Per Cent Absent	Total WTE Absent	Total Per cent Absent
		Uncert.	Self Cert.	Med. Cert.		Ann. Leave	Bank Hol.	Auth.	Un-auth.	Mat Leave	Inserv. Train.	Other Train.			
Physio	34.99	.64	.04	.04	2.06	5.26	3.17	.05				.63	26.04	9.83	28.
Phy. Help	7.11	.17			2.39	.64	.77	.26				.15	25.60	1.99	27.
Total	42.10	.81	.04	.04	2.22	5.90	3.94	.31	.00	.00		.78	25.82	11.82	27.50

Figures are in Monthly Whole Time Equivalents.
Source of Absence Information: Timesheets and Timecards.
Source of Staff in Post Information: Payroll (Cost Centres).

Figure 7.1. Summary of staff absences—April 1990

The National Return for physiotherapy (KT27) requires that the sample should be used to analyse the pattern of work. The information required to be collected by physiotherapists includes details of the exact time spent on a variety of specified activities during the sample period. Physiotherapists are *not* required to collect data on 'face-to-face' contacts with patients on a daily basis. The sample inquiry information to be collected is:

1 face-to-face contacts;
2 telephone contacts with patients or relatives;
3 home assessment visits—this does not mean domiciliary physiotherapy treatments;
4 other professional activities.

It is desirable to break these four rather broad and vague data items down further, in order to give a more detailed picture of physiotherapists' activity locally. This will probably also be more acceptable to physiotherapists who feel that the four broad categories required nationally do not meaningfully reflect their daily work patterns.

Figure 7.2 represents one possible form design for the collection of the sample inquiry data. This form allows for the collection of the national Körner requirements and data which will be useful to Physiotherapy Managers and clinicians locally. All staff members complete a form each day of the survey period. It may not be necessary to complete the left side of the form—'Initial Contacts (New Patients Today)' and 'All Other Contacts

DISTRICT PHYSIOTHERAPY SERVICE

Sample Inquiry

DATE						SITE	CLINICIAN	GRADE	POST

INITIAL CONTACTS (NEW PATIENTS TODAY)

PATIENT		SOURCE OF REFERRAL	SEX	YEAR OF BIRTH	LOCATION	GROUP	HELPER ALONE	DOUBLE	TREBLE
IN	OUT								

ALL OTHER CONTACTS (TODAY)

ACTIVITY LEVEL

	HOURS	MINS
FACE TO FACE CONTACTS (INDIVIDUAL)		
FACE TO FACE CONTACTS (GROUP)		
TELEPHONE CONTACTS PATIENT OR RELATIVE		
WARD ROUNDS		
CASE CONFERENCE		
STUDY LEAVE		
LIAISON WITH OTHER SERVICES		
ADMINISTRATION		
MANAGEMENT DUTIES		
HOME ASSESSMENT VISITS		
TRAVEL		
CLINICS		
STAFF/TEAM MEETINGS		
IN-SERVICE TRAINING		
TEACHING PHYSIO'S		
TEACHING STUDENTS		
TEACHING HEALTH PROF'S		
TEACHING PUBLIC		
CLINICAL SUPERVISION		
OTHER		
TIME TAKEN TO COMPLETE THIS FORM		
NORMAL WORKING HOURS		

No. OF GROUP SESSIONS TODAY	
No. OF HOME ASSESSMENT VISITS THIS QUARTER	
TOTAL CASELOAD	

REASON FOR ABSENCE		

Figure 7.2.   The sample inquiry form

(Today)'—this will be dependent on the computer system, if any, in use within the physiotherapy service. Physiotherapy helpers complete only the top and right side of the form as they do not carry clinical responsibility for a case-load; this responsibility is carried by qualified staff.

Notes on the sample inquiry form

Each member of staff completes a new form on each sample inquiry day. The form divides into three sections. At the top:

- date of sample;
- site—where the staff member works;
- clinician–physiotherapist identifier code;
- helpers also identify themselves in these boxes;
- grade—of staff member;
- post—indicates placement in the case of rotational posts.

The right side of the form deals with the allocation of time throughout the day.

The left side of the form provides for the recording of information about new patients on the day of the sample inquiry and also the on-going patients seen that day. In physiotherapy services where there are computer systems handling information about patient episodes of care, it may not be necessary to use the left side of the form. In these instances, the patient registration and de-registration details will provide this information.

Analysis of the pattern of work

For the purposes of the National KT27 Return, the data items listed on the sample inquiry form may be aggregated into the four categories required by the DoH:

1 face-to-face contacts;
2 telephone contacts with patients or relatives;
3 home assessment visits;
4 other professional activities.

However, the sample inquiry form used as an example here provides a much more detailed breakdown of activities. The computer readouts below are examples of statistical and bar-chart presentations of information from the sample inquiry. There are several ways of presenting this information, but the use of a computerized system is essential to the whole process.

The data made available through this method of sample inquiry are likely to be helpful in the costing and pricing procedures which will be necessary

Physiotherapy System

Sample Data Report

Data collected on 22 March 1990

Totals and % of time spent in hours and minutes for:

		Total	% of Actual Time
Individual Face to Face Contacts	:	139:26	46.8%
Group Face to Face Contacts	:	28:25	9.5%
Telephone	:	3:59	1.3%
Ward Rounds	:	5:00	1.6%
Case Conference	:	1:35	0.5%
Study Leave	:	5:00	1.6%
Liaison	:	12:09	4.0%
Admin.	:	37:37	12.6%
Management	:	9.34	3.2%
Home Assessment Visits	:	1:15	0.4%
Travel	:	12:59	4.3%
Clinics	:	0:50	0.2%
Staff/Team Meeting	:	6:55	2.3%
In Service Training	:	0:00	0.0%
Teaching – Physios	:	0:10	0.0%
– Students	:	3:35	1.2%
– Health Professional	:	0:20	0.1%
– Public	:	1:00	0.3%
Clinical Supervision	:	1:15	0.4%
Other	:	18:35	6.2%
Time Taken to Complete this Form	:	7:41	2.5%
Standard Working Day (Totals)	:	330:15	0.0%
Actual Time Spent	:	297:20	

Total number of home assessment visits this **quarter** :   9

No. of group sessions today :   16

Total caseload :   996

End of Report

Figure 7.3.   Sample inquiry data report in statistical presentation

in the context of RMI and contracts. The four data items required in the national return are of very limited value in this respect. There are a variety of other possible uses for the information collected in this sort of sample inquiry. Physiotherapy Managers will be able to use the data in, for example, service planning, audit, and quality assurance including efficiency indicators, monitoring and costing.

Figures 7.3 and 7.4 are examples of a survey taken on one sample inquiry day. It may be useful to undertake this on one day each quarter of the year to gain a more complete picture of work patterns.

Figure 7.5 is a bar-chart showing a comparison between the results of two sample inquiry days.

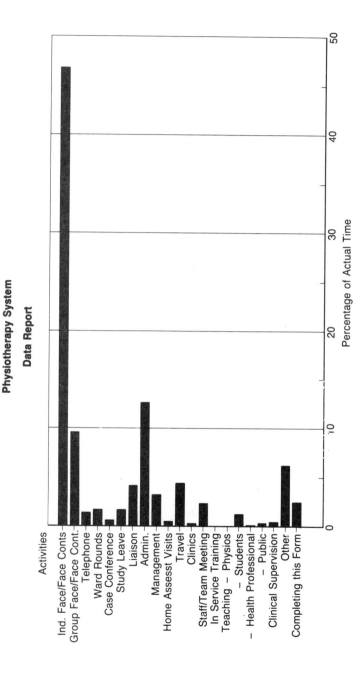

Figure 7.4.   Sample inquiry data report in bar-chart presentation

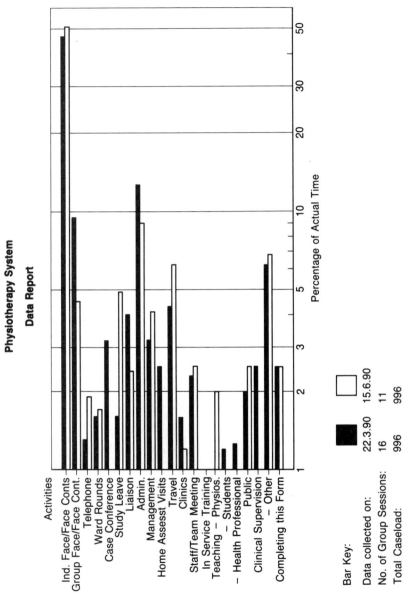

Figure 7.5. Comparison sample inquiry data reports—two inquiry days

The Körner minimum data set

The Körner Reports criticized the old SH3 method of statistical returns on several grounds and recommended the introduction of a 'minimum data set' (MDS) for the PAMs. The Fourth Körner Report states: 'we have not succeeded in identifying data which adequately reflect the work done by staff in these disciplines' (Körner 1985).[1] However, Körner recommended that the MDS should include:

- A count (1 April to 31 March) of the number of physiotherapy episodes of care begun in the year—'initial contacts'.
- A count of the 'first contacts in the financial year'. This figure will represent the total number of people who have had contact with the physiotherapy service during the financial year, however many episodes they may have had.
- The initial contacts are categorized by sex, age and source of referral.
- First contacts are summarized by age and sex and the use of physiotherapy time (*see* sample inquiry above and Figure 7.6 the DoH Return, Form KT27).

Physiotherapy patient registration document

The South East Thames Regional Health Authority Physiotherapy Information Systems and Resource Management Group developed a multi-purpose patient registration document that would:

1 fulfil DoH, RHA and DHA requirements;
2 facilitate the registration of patients coming into contact with the physiotherapy service;
3 enable registration of information at the conclusion of the episode of care;
4 be used as a patient referral card;
5 provide for POMRs;
6 provide for the collection of other useful information;
7 all these purposes to be incorporated in one document in order to control the volume of paperwork for physiotherapy clinicians.

The system described here is one approach to a method of recording data and it is fully acknowledged that there may be different and equally acceptable and efficient ways of achieving a satisfactory result.

The data collection element of the document is a three-piece NCR (self-carboning) section, of which the top two parts are detachable. The detachable slips are the patient registration discharge computer input forms, while the third part is the top section of the POMR card (*see* Figure 7.7).

DHSS Form KT27

Year ending March 19 [   ]　　　Quarter　　1　　2　　3　　4

District/SHA Code [   ]　　　Name [   ]

Part 1 Initial Contacts – Source of Referral

Source of Referral	Code	Total number of initial contacts
Hospital specialties		
Trauma and Orthopaedics	110	
General medicine	300	
Geriatric medicine	430	
Mental handicap	700	
Mental illness	710	
Other (specify and use codes in Appendix C)		
General practice	010	
Other medical	020	
Self referral	030	
Other sources	099	
Total	9999	

0451d/19/31-22

Part 2A　Initial Contacts – Age and Sex of Patients

Note: This part to be provided only by authorities not producing Part 2B

Sex		Age 0 – 4	5 – 15	16 – 54	55 – 64	65 – 74	75 – 84	85 and over	Total all ages
Male	0001								
Female	0002								
Total	9999								

Figure 7.6. Form KT27, summary of physiotherapy services

Part 2B Initial Contacts – Age, Sex and Source of Referral

Note: This part to be provided by authorities with computerised, patient – based systems for 1988/89 and by all authorities for 1989/90 onwards.

Source of referral	Males – age 0–4	5–15	16–54	55–64	65–74	75–84	85 and over	Males Total all ages
Hospital specialties								
Surgical group 0001								
Medical group 0002								
Psychiatry group 0003								
Other 0004								
Other sources 0005								
Total 0006								

Source of referral	Females – age 0–4	5–15	16–54	55–64	65–74	75–84	85 and over	Females Total all ages
Hospital specialties								
Surgical group 0007								
Medical Group 0008								
Psychiatry group 0009								
Other 0010								
Other sources 0011								
Total 0012								

Part 3 First Contacts – Age and Sex of Patients

Sex	Age 0–4	5–15	16–54	55–64	65–74	75–84	85 and over	Total all ages
Male 0001								
Female 0002								
Total 9999								

Part 4 Results of Survey of Activity Year End Only

Type of activity	Percentage of time (nearest whole number)
Face-to-face contacts 0001	
Telephone contacts 0002	
Home assessment visits 0003	
Other professional acitivity 0004	
Total	100

Part 5 Home Assessment Visits

Total Number	9999	

0451d/22/44-2

Figure 7.6. continued

PHYSIOTHERAPY PATIENT REGISTRATION

REFERRAL DATE		NHS	PP	OSV	SSC		ID												HOSPITAL No.		
							MR		SURNAME												
FIRST PHYSIOTHERAPY APPT.		CLASSIFICATION					MRS MISS							SEX		DOB				
		A&E	IP	OP	COM	DAY	FORENAMES													
DIAGNOSTIC CODE							ADDRESS				GP						
		LOCATION															
REF. SOURCE	CONSULTANT	REASON FOR REF.	WEIGHTING								No.						
							POSTCODE			TEL: HOME			WORK		
DISCHARGE DATE		DISCHARGE STATUS				OUTCOME MEASURES					No. of HAVS	APPLIANCES		CLINICIAN
TOTAL CONTACTS		PRIU						AUDIT					
CLINIC FOLLOW-UP APPT.		CONSULTANT			OCCUPATION				HOSPITAL TRANSPORT	CAR		WALKER
										CHAIR		STRETCHER

REFERRED BY:

DIAGNOSIS & DATE OF ONSET:

X-RAY REPORT:

MEDICATION:

RELEVANT MEDICAL HISTORY:

PHYSIOTHERAPY DISCHARGE SUMMARY

SIGNATURE

Figure 7.7. Patient registration document—the computer input section

The data items—registration

The following items are entered when the patient is referred into the physiotherapy service:

(a)   referral date.

(b)   first physiotherapy appointment—from which the computer will sort 'initial contact' and 'first contacts' in the financial year (see above). The difference between (a) and (b) will give waiting times.

(c)   diagnostic code.

(d)   referral source and consultant codes.

(e)   NHS, PP, OSV—National Health Service patient, private patient, or overseas visitor.

(f)   SSC—social support code (this may be used to indicate where a patient is receiving support from other services).

(g)   classification—A&E, IP, OP, COM, DAY (this shows whether the patient was referred from Accident and Emergency, In-patient, Out-patient, Community or Day facility).

(h)   location code—indicates where the patient has physiotherapy, for example, a DGH Physiotherapy Out-patient Department or in the patient's own home.

(i)   reason for referral—this refers to the 'physiotherapy reason for referral' and not necessarily the medical diagnosis. Alternatively, these boxes might be used for some method of case-weighting. At present, there are no universally accepted methods of coding and recording physiotherapy reasons for referral. However, as the *Clinical and Managerial Information Systems for Physiotherapy and Occupational Therapy Report* (CSP/COT/DHSS 1982)[2] suggests, it is also appropriate to know the physiotherapy reason for referral as well as the medical diagnosis.

(j)   weighting—this may be necessary if (i) is used for 'Physiotherapy reason for referral'.

(k)   ID—these boxes may be used for a personal identifier code or for another form of identification such as the patient's NHS number.

(l)   name, address, post code, hospital number, sex, date of birth, general practitioner code and patient's telephone number. This personal details section is designed to enable the use of PAS-type labelling where available.

(m)   clinician—these boxes are for the physiotherapy clinician code. Codes may be developed locally to represent the physiotherapist, where that person works and his grade. It is possible to incorporate all this information in a three-box code.

The top slip is detached and submitted to the physiotherapy computer officer for entry.

The data items—discharge

(a) Discharge date.

(b) Total contacts—this is the total number of contacts with the service during the physiotherapy episode of care.

(c) Discharge status—this code may indicate, for example, whether the patient is discharged to another district, another condition intervened, discharge fully recovered and so on.

(d) PRIU (Physiotherapy Resource Input Unit)—these boxes may be used to indicate some measure of physiotherapy resource input during the physiotherapy episode of care (see below).

(e) Outcome measure—there are a variety of methods by which this might be coded.

(f) Audit—codes may be devised to facilitate clinical audit.

(g) Number of HAVs—refers to home assessment visits (not domiciliary physiotherapy treatments).

(h) Appliances—coding to be used for recording and retrieval of appliances, and equipment loaned or provided.

The discharge section of the second slip is completed when the patient concludes the physiotherapy episode of care. This is then submitted to the computer officer for entry into the system.

The data items—POMR

This section comprises a four-sided POMR and referral card. Side one contains the self-carbonated information from the registration and discharge slips, the referral details (*see* Figure 7.7) and the physiotherapist's discharge summary are also entered on the front of the document. Sides two, three and four comprise the standard POMR format.

Statistics and reports

There are two main types of computer reports which are 'Standard' and 'Ad hoc' reports. Standard reports are pre-defined at the time the computer programme is written, while ad hoc reports allow the user to choose or mix and match a variety of criteria. For national and regional statistical returns, the computer system should generate a number of standard reports. An example of this is the KT27 national return, 'Summary of Physiotherapy Services', which should be programmed into the computer system as a standard report so that the information is available from the system very quickly and without having to ask the computer a detailed series of questions. The information for this particular report is calculated by the computer on an 'on-going' basis so that a print out can be taken off the printer when required as a result of a single computer command. Another example of a standard report is the Körner sample inquiry data (*see* Figures 7.3 and 7.4). Other standard reports may be programmed into the system as required for local needs.

The ad hoc reporting facility allows search and extract from the database, that is, from the range of data input on patient registration and discharge slips. Some examples of ad hoc reports which might be printed out are:

- individual patient reports;
- the number of 'open' and 'closed' episodes of care;
- patient age ranges;
- waiting times;
- staff case-loads;
- comparison of case-load by sources of referral;
- patient classification;
- diagnosis or reasons for referral;
- outcomes and audit information;
- referrals classified by individual or groups of consultants;
- proportion of GP referrals;
- number of patients referred by particular GP practices;
- appliances provided and for retrieval.

There are many other possible questions which might be asked using an ad hoc reporting facility. Any such queries might be made in isolation or in combination with other questions. An example of this would be to ask the computer how many patients over the age of 65 years were referred from Consultant 'A' with a certain diagnosis, and treated in a particular location. Alternatively, a report may be needed on the number of patients referred from a particular GP practice or simply the number of self-referrals.

Values may be presented as proportions or numbers of the database, or in percentages. It should also be possible to move information across from the database into spreadsheet or graphics presentations (*see* Chapter 8). Therefore, the data can be printed in a variety of ways to suit the particular purpose.

Response times on ad hoc and standard report production should be minimal. It is important that computer print-outs are obtainable almost immediately from the system on request as delay may render the data useless or meaningless, and users will quickly become disillusioned. It is unacceptable, and very frustrating, for Physiotherapy Managers to have to wait several weeks, or even months, for specific information.

In order to be effective, there are several requirements relating to data and reporting systems which must be satisfied. These may be summarized as the 'five As' and the 'five Fs'.

Data must be:

1 Accurate
2 Accessible
3 Acceptable
4 Adequate
5 Appropriate

Reporting systems must be:

1 Flexible
2 Fault-free
3 Failure-free
4 Frequent
5 Foolproof!

An example of a standard report is that shown in Figure 7.3, 'Sample inquiry data report'. Examples of ad hoc reports are shown below in a variety of formats including statistical, bar-charts and pie-charts. These are Figures 7.8 – 7.14(b).

. . . Health Authority			
1989		**1990**	
Jan	154 patients	Jan	211 patients
Feb	144 patients	Feb	150 patients
Mar	154 patients	Mar	205 patients
Apr	160 patients	Apr	184 patients
May	136 patients		
June	119 patients		
Jul	147 patients		
Aug	123 patients		
Sept	97 patients		
Oct	217 patients		
Nov	177 patients		
Dec	160 patients		

Figure 7.8. New referrals to the DGH Physiotherapy Out-patient Department in numerical presentation—January 1989 to April 1990

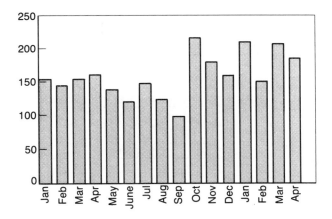

Figure 7.9. New referrals to the DGH Physiotherapy Out-patient Department in bar-chart presentation—January 1989 to April 1990

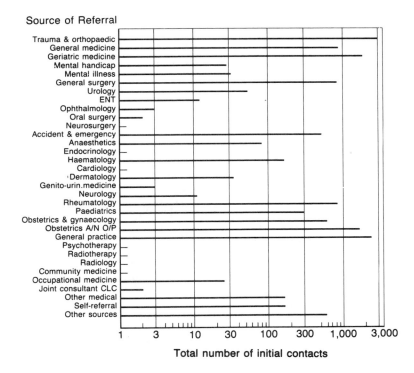

Figure 7.10. Sources of referrral to physiotherapy—taken from KT27, 31 March 1990

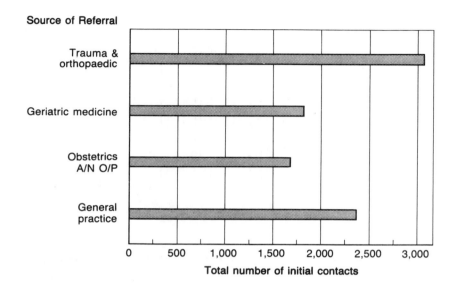

Figure 7.11. Sources of referral to physiotherapy—the top four users by number of referrals, 1 April 1989 to 31 March 1990

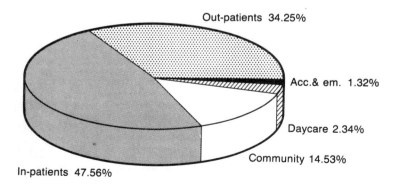

Figure 7.12. Physiotherapy episodes of care by classification, 1 April 1989 to 31 March 1990

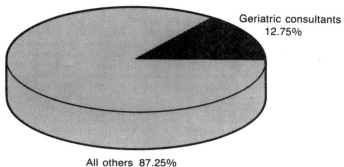

Geriatric consultants
12.75%

All others 87.25%

Figure 7.13. Total numbers of patients referred to physiotherapy by the three geriatricians—an analysis of service use over one year, 1 April 1989 to 31 March 1990

CONSULTANTS

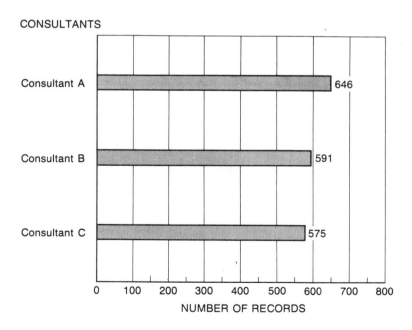

Figure 7.14(a). Comparison of consultant use of physiotherapy services—the three geriatricians, 1 April 1989 to 31 March 1990

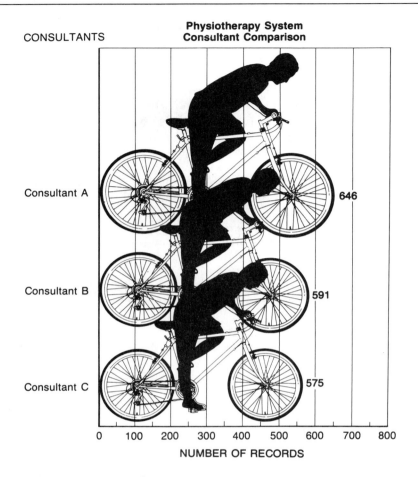

Figure 7.14(b).   As Figure 7.14(a)—a pictorial presentation!

Körner requirement information for national purposes has been found to be of little or no use centrally, or regionally. However, much of the information will be of value locally.

Performance indicators

Performance indicators in the NHS are sets of statistics which allow comparisons to be made between the Districts. 'Indicators are measurements of service provision and effectiveness designed to permit comparison between the health services of different health Districts and to stimulate local enquiry about how effectively those services are being delivered' (DoH 1990)[3].

The performance indicators are issued in the form of a floppy disk by the DoH, well after the year to which they refer. The DoH has recently reviewed the performance indicators, and those recommended for physiotherapy services are as follows:

- PY41, Source KT27—first contacts at any location related to age groups; 0–4, 5–15 and 75 + in the District resident population.
- PY42, Source KT27—number of first contacts by physiotherapists with persons aged 75 + and children aged 0–4 and 5–15 in a non-hospital location related to the District resident population aged 75 + and children aged 0–4 and 5–15.
- PY42 also to include—number of first contacts by physiotherapy staff with patients aged 16–64 in non-hospital locations, related to District resident population aged 16–64 (if the indicator of the contribution of physiotherapists to services which allow those younger disabled people with severe disabilities to live in ordinary housing is to be introduced, a change will be necessary to the KT27 return).

Manpower indicators

- PY22—total staff per first contacts.
- PY34—percentage qualified physiotherapists of total physiotherapy staff.
- PY23—qualified physiotherapy staff per resident population.

A further physiotherapy indicator is PY01 which gives the net cost of physiotherapy to resident population.

Definitions

- First contact—the first face-to-face contact in the District after 31 March each year.
- Initial contact—the first face-to-face contact of an episode of care.

The performance indicators PY23—qualified physiotherapists per 100,000 District resident population—and PY34—percentage of qualified physiotherapists of total physiotherapy staff—are shown in Figures 7.15 and 7.16. These indicators show Districts grouped together in bandings of similar value. On the examples here, the Districts in the South East Thames RHA are identified.

The DoH Performance Indicator Working Group have placed the onus for developing further meaningful performance indicators in the hands of the PAMs themselves: 'The responsibility remains with the professions concerned to propose indicators which more closely reflect the results of their work, both with individual patients and as advisers to other carers' (DoH 1990).[4]

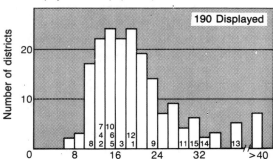

Qual. physio.: res. pop. for prof. allied to medicine 1988

Number of qualified physiotherapists per 100,000
District resident population

0 Zero values;	0 Excluded;	0 Missing;	8 No service
1 Brighton	2 Eastbourne		3 Hastings
4 South East Kent	5 Canterbury		6 Dartford
7 Maidstone	8 Medway		9 Tunbridge Wells
10 Bexley	11 Greenwich		12 Bromley
13 West Lambeth	14 Camberwell		15 Lewisham

exc Excluded values, mis Missing data, nos No service

PY23 Qualified physiotherapists: resident population
   Qualified physiotherapists per 100,000 District resident population
* NUMERATOR: Number of qualified physiotherapists (contract hours WTE) in
   District at 30 September.
   Source: NMM Census
   DENOMINATOR: Total estimated resident population in District at 30
   September.
   Source: OPCS population data

Figure 7.15.   Health Service indicators. Qualified physiotherapy staff per 100,000 resident
population

Introduction to resource management

Background

Notice that resource management was to be introduced into the NHS was
given by the NHS Finance Director in HN(86)34 *Resource Management
(Management Budgeting) for Health Authorities* (DHSS 1986).[5] The aims
of resource management as set out in HN(86)34 were: 'To enable the NHS
to give a better service by helping clinicians and other managers make better
informed judgements about how the resources they control can be used to

% qual. physio. for prof.. allied to medicine 1988

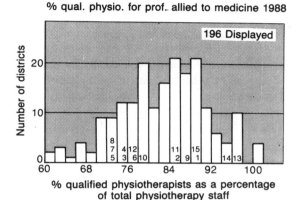

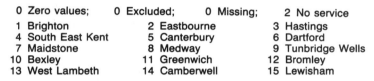

0 Zero values;   0 Excluded;   0 Missing;   2 No service

1 Brighton	2 Eastbourne	3 Hastings
4 South East Kent	5 Canterbury	6 Dartford
7 Maidstone	8 Medway	9 Tunbridge Wells
10 Bexley	11 Greenwich	12 Bromley
13 West Lambeth	14 Camberwell	15 Lewisham

exc Excluded values, mis Missing data, nos No service

PY34 Qualified as % of physiotherapy staff
Qualified physiotherapists as a percentage of total physiotherapy staff
* NUMERATOR: Number of qualified physiotherapists (contract hours plus worked hours WTE for bank/agency staff) in District at September.
Source: NMM Census, MDS
DENOMINATOR: Total number of physiotherapy staff (contract hours plus worked hours WTE for bank/agency staff) in District at September.
Source: NMM Census, MDS

Figure 7.16.   Health Service indicators. Qualified physiotherapists as a percentage of total physiotherapy staff

the maximum effect'. The system proposed before resource management was management budgeting, a budget setting and costing system only. Clinical matters were not within the remit of management budgeting and for this reason the experiment failed due to lack of support from clinicians in all disciplines. Resource management, on the other hand, recognizes the importance of providing clinicians with clinical information.

The NHS Management Executive defines resource management as, a complex process with a single aim—to allow total, individual, high quality patient care to be planned, delivered and costed more effectively'

DoH 1990).[6] This definition is rooted in the 1986 Health Notice from which a number of subsidiary objectives may be drawn. These include the provision for clinicians of information which enables them to:

- identify areas of waste and inefficiency;
- benefit from clinical group discussions and review;
- highlight areas which could most benefit from more resources;
- identify and expose the health care consequences of given financial policies and constraints;
- understand the comparative costs of future health care options and hold informed debates about such options (IBM 1990).[7]

Resource management was started during 1986 in six large acute hospitals as a pilot project. Following on from this, Mr Roger Freeman, the then Parliamentary Under-Secretary of State for Health, announced in March 1989 the names of 50 further hospitals which were to be supported by the NHS Executive in starting up resource management projects. The aim of the NHS Management Executive is to have all 260 large acute hospitals embarked upon the main phase of the RMI by 1993. Clearly, therefore, resource management will impact on all physiotherapy services in a variety of ways by that time at the latest. Resource management includes all aspects of service provision and hospital activity, and it is likely that community services will also be included formally within the next few years as service specifications and contracts are developed.

In 1987, a number of main features of resource management in the six acute hospital pilot sites were identified (Williams 1987).[8]

- Speciality and consultant costing systems in detail.
- Development of case mix measures for planning and management purposes.
- The development of advanced nursing dependency and management systems.
- Linked financial and staff activity systems.
- Future budget setting based on planned activity levels and case-mix costs.
- Regular report generation and on-going monitoring against budgets and planned activity.
- The development of costing systems.
- Comparison of actual and predicted use of resources to allow monitoring of clinical performance and deployment of resources.

The main features of resource management projects in 1990 include all of these, some of them expressed in different ways. There is now particular emphasis on:

- development of costing mechanisms;
- development of pricing mechanisms for contract purposes;

- development of care profiles for clinical and managerial audit purposes;
- the installation of case-mix systems and computers;
- coding systems;
- balancing organizational development and clinical information systems.

These lists of work areas do not completely indicate what is involved in RMIs because projects vary greatly in methodology and systems deployment from one District to another. Again, there is no right or only one way of doing it. The lists indicate simply the main areas of activity with RMI projects. The development of appropriate and relevant information systems in physiotherapy will be crucial to the way in which the RMI impacts upon physiotherapy services and also what physiotherapy services will be able to gain from RMI projects themselves. For this reason, the Physiotherapy Manager will need a clear understanding of, and willingness to participate in, the development of RMI projects locally.

Case-mix management

Case-mix management systems (CMMS) are computerized information systems which are central to the development of RMI projects. Such systems must satisfy the core specification laid down by the NHS Management Executive Resource Management Unit as well as local needs. 'CMMS is a system which provides a common management information data base to clinicians and managers as an aid to improve effective and efficient use of resources and measurable improvements in patient care' (R.M. Directorate, DoH, 1989).[9]

The basis of case-mix systems is a record of every patient which includes information about every event occurring during a complete episode of hospital care. Such a record includes the patient's personal details, diagnoses and operative procedures, together with all diagnostic events and therapeutic interventions, for example, X-rays, blood tests, drugs or physiotherapy episodes of care. All of these events have resource use implications in manpower, materials, facilities and so on. Therefore, costing is an element of the case-mix equation.

Detailed information will be available from case-mix systems for clinical audit, quality control and clinical research, as well as for resource use, which includes mechanisms for costing and pricing. Information about care profiles against which actual care can be compared is held in the CMMS. These care profiles may relate to groups of patients under the care of individual doctors. It would also be possible to include various care profiles for physiotherapy if this were desirable. CMMS will facilitate detailed reporting, analysis and presentation of a wide range of data. It will also enable individual professional staff and managers to obtain information for their own purposes within the service.

The computerized CMMS or so-called 'black, central, or big box' will receive data from a wide range of operational feeder systems throughout the local service. Patient identification and details of hospital stay will typically be downloaded to the CMMS from the PAS. Other events will be downloaded to the CMMS by the individual operational computer feeder systems throughout the hospital. Computerized physiotherapy information systems should be able to download agreed information to the case-mix system in their own right. In *Resource Management Initiative, Technical Guidance Notes—for roll-out sites* (DoH 1989),[10] the Resource Management Directorate cites certain operational systems as being 'essential' for effective resource management, these are:

- patient administration systems;
- nursing systems, and any two out of:
    pathology,
    radiology,
    pharmacy and
    operating theatres.

However the document also lists physiotherapy as a service which will be part of the CMMS.

It will be necessary for the Physiotherapy Manager to agree locally the data items which are relevant to the case-mix system and also the information required for use within the physiotherapy service. It is likely that only a limited number of data items will be required for the CMMS. Physiotherapy Managers and clinicians will also want some information from the case-mix system and this too will need to be agreed locally. It is essential that the computerized physiotherapy information system provides operational benefit to the physiotherapy service as well as data items for the case-mix system. If the physiotherapy information system is perceived as being of use to physiotherapy itself, the accuracy of the data is more likely to be assured.

Figure 7.17 represents diagrammatically one possible configuration of a case-mix system.

Coding

The NHS uses a variety of coding systems:

- HIPE—hospital in-patient enquiry, a one in 10 sample of information about hospital in-patients;
- HAA—hospital activity analysis, this is a comprehensive data set;
- Körner—minimum data sets from a wide range of services, including physiotherapy.

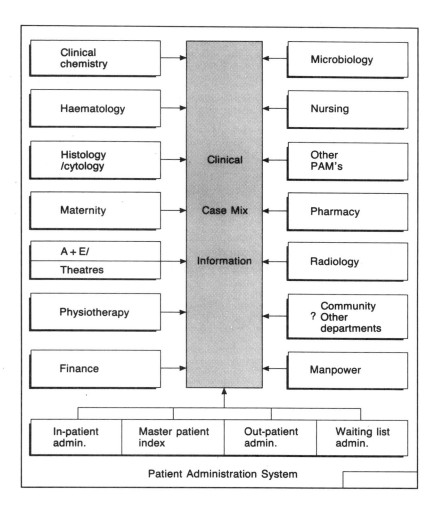

Figure 7.17. Resource management project information systems

The object of coding systems must be to provide a common and shared factual basis or language which can be used both by clinicians from all disciplines and managers. There are six 'key criteria' which a 'standard computerized medical language must satisfy' (Read & Benson 1986).[11] The language must be:

1 comprehensive;
2 hierarchical;
3 computerized;

4 coded;
5 cross-referenced;
6 dynamic.

James Read has developed a clinical classification system which fulfils all of these criteria and which is likely to be used by many Health Authorities in conjunction with resource management projects.

Coding systems currently used in the NHS which may be of particular relevance to physiotherapy include ICD-9—International Classification of Diseases, 9th revision and OPCS-4—Classification of Surgical Operations and Procedures, 4th revision. On the question of coding for patient identification, the DoH is now recommending the use of the patient's NHS number as the 'universal patient identifier'. This will come into use by 1 April 1993 (DoH 1990).[12]

There are currently several coding methods in use in conjunction with physiotherapy information systems in different parts of the country. Some of these systems use codes for data items such as physiotherapy reasons for referral, outcomes, physiotherapy clinicians and appliances loaned to patients. At present, there is no national coding system.

Diagnosis related groups (DRGs)

Diagnosis related groups were first proposed in the United States by Professor Bob Fetter of Yale University (DoH 1989).[13] This is a method of grouping clinically similar patients in order to support quality control systems in hospitals. The DRG classifications contain 470 such groups. DRGs are also used in some places in the United States as a finance or costing tool. Although they were originally recommended as a method of grouping patient data in the six original NHS resource management pilot sites (DHSS 1986),[14] the use of DRGs in this country is now the subject of some debate.

Developments in data requirements for physiotherapy

In January 1990, a set of three consultative documents entitled *Framework for Information Systems* was published by the DoH. Working Paper 11 was an overview, while the other two were on information technology and information (DoH 1990).[15] There were 13 individual annexes associated with the paper on information.

Following the consultation process for these documents, the DoH published, during June 1990, *Framework for Information Systems: The Next Steps* (DoH 1990).[16] This has a very wide-ranging content on most aspects of information within the NHS; Section 15 relates to so-called 'paramedical services', which include physiotherapy.

In summary, Sections 15 and 50 acknowledge that the changes required in information systems under the Körner recommendations for the PAMs were not yet complete in all areas. These systems were supposed to have been in place from 1 April 1988. For this reason substantial changes are not now proposed until 1 April 1991. 'Thus for 1991 the provider and contract mds will, in essence, be Körner' (DoH 1990)[17] (mds = minimum data set).

Alteration to the definition of 'First Contacts' is proposed because of the changes in health care provision resulting from the Government's NHS reforms.

'Körner incorporated the concept of first contact in the financial year, and initial contact, in the District. This concept will need to change to first contact in the financial year, and initial contact, with the provider' (DoH 1990).[18] This means that episodes of care will in future relate to providers rather than to districts.

The *Next Steps* document will undoubtedly impact on physiotherapy in a variety of ways. However, there is not space here to discuss these in detail, merely to point the direction. The paper merits deeper study in its own right.

Costing and pricing of physiotherapy services

Before the advent of Körner and the introduction of computerized information systems into physiotherapy services little work on costing and pricing physiotherapy in the NHS was undertaken. There are several reasons why work in this area is now happening with increasing urgency in many parts of the country. Some of these influences are: the imperative laid down by the Government to provide value for money and be able to demonstrate this, the requirement for effective and efficient service provision, the greater availability of reliable data and an increasing awareness of data use by Physiotherapy Managers and the Government reforms of the NHS. These recently enacted health service reforms (*see* Chapter 5), under which Health Authorities will purchase services from a variety of providers, further increases the urgency for sound costing and pricing mechanisms to be instituted. As a result of all of these, and other factors, Physiotherapy Managers will undoubtedly become increasingly involved in this field.

An essential requirement for the design and operation of a sound costing and pricing system will be a computerized information system. It will need to be comprehensive, dynamic, effective and efficient, with the properties outlined in 'main factors for consideration in physiotherapy information systems design' and 'statistics and reports'—the five As and Fs' (*see* page 76). It may be that some purchasing authorities and provider units will decide that it is easier to cost and price physiotherapy services as overheads to larger service contracts. However, meaningful physiotherapy costing and pricing mechanisms will provide a further opportunity for physiotherapy services to be recognized in their own right for the contribution they make to overall health care provision and in a system where 'money follows patients' this should be a positive step for the service. There are also some instances in which it will be necessary for contracts specific to physiotherapy itself to be drawn up. An example of this is GP open access to physiotherapy out-patient departments. A physiotherapy pricing mechanism will also be required by those Physiotherapy Managers who are embarking on selling services to non-NHS purchasers in the wider community.

Many of the tools needed for costing and pricing physiotherapy services are already available for Physiotherapy Managers, although even in those Districts with comprehensive information systems there is still a great deal of work to be done. As yet, there is no universally agreed method of costing and pricing, but helpful proposals on possible ways of approaching this problem are now beginning to emerge from several locations around the country.

A first step is to examine the data already available so as to establish what information will be of use for the process. Through this approach, it will become apparent what necessary information is missing from the equation and where further development work must take place.

Definitions

Some basic definitions may be helpful in the further discussion of these financial matters.

- Cost—this is taken to mean the expenditure incurred to produce goods or provide a service. The cost to the NHS of providing a service must take into account expenditure on work-force, equipment, drugs, facilities and various overheads. The cost of a service to a buyer is a measurement in cash terms of what that purchaser has to part with in order to obtain that service. When a service provider sells a service to a purchaser, he will normally sell at the price sufficient to cover his full costs plus profit, where that is appropriate.
- Costing—this is the system by which the cost of service provision is calculated.
- Marginal cost—the additional cost incurred by producing just one more unit of production, or treating just one more patient.
- Variable costs—those costs which vary according to the level of activity, for example, materials.
- Fixed costs—these are the costs which do not vary when activity increases or decreases. In some respects, pay costs are fixed in terms of physiotherapy services because of manpower and contract constraints. However, these costs may vary marginally in terms of, for example, 'on-call' services and overtime. In the almost unprecedented event of workloads decreasing, staff vacancies arising may not be filled; in such circumstances, pay would not be a fixed cost.

- Price—the amount at which a service is valued, bought or sold. A measure of what a purchaser must expend in order to obtain the service.
- Overheads—those expenses incurred by the service provider over and above the direct cost of providing the service itself and the materials associated with this. Examples of such indirect costs would be building maintenance and administration.
- Standard costs—these are planned target costs for an area of activity or unit of production, for example, a standard cost per case could be calculated, assuming the average costs incurred in treating a certain type of case. In practice, the actual cost of treating each case may turn out to be more, or less, than the pre-calculated standard.

What information is already available?

A variety of essential information for costing and pricing is available in all Districts.

(a) Budget statements

These give a breakdown of the total financial allocation to the physiotherapy service for the year. Budget allocation and expenditure to date are stated in the areas of staff pay, equipment, travel, appliances, consumables and services provided, etc. This information relates to the financial cost of providing the service and is vital to the costing/pricing of physiotherapy.

(b) Körner 3—Manpower information (see 'Körner requirements' page 62)

These data are collected by all DHAs and relate to the amount of time which staff are absent from work and the nature of such absences, that is, annual leave, sickness, maternity leave, study leave, and so on. When all of these and other absence factors are taken into account, a physiotherapist might be expected to be actually in the work-place for approximately 40–42 weeks of the year. This will be an important part of the financial equation.

(c) The Körner sample inquiry data (see 'Physiotherapy staff activity—the sample inquiry' page 62)

Figures 7.3, 7.4 and 7.5 are examples of the sort of information which can be obtained. On average, physiotherapists typically spend between 55 and 65% of their time in 'face-to-face' or 'hands-on' contact with patients. This is another important factor in the financial calculation of cost and price. Under the provisions of the NHS and Community Care Act (1990)—health service reforms—money will follow patients. It will, therefore, be necessary to know the proportion of total staff time spent in face-to-face contact, proxy contact (patient-related activity) and non-patient-related activity. Costing mechanisms will need to take the percentages into account.

(d) Data about the patients using the service—KT27, 'Summary of Physiotherapy Services' and 'Patient Registration Document' (see page 69)

Full details of the information required for the KT27 return are given on page 73. The information relating to numbers of episodes of care provided in relation to sources of referral may be used to proportion the volume of work to specialities, GP practices, self-referral and so on.

(e) Staff information

Physiotherapy Managers will have available to them a full list of their staff, including grade mix, again an important part of the equation.

Such staff as some Senior Physiotherapy Managers, clerical and secretarial officers, porters and others do not carry responsibility for a case-load. Such details will be required for the apportionment of these staff costs into the physiotherapy prices.

(f) Capital charges

Under the provisions of the NHS and Community Care Act (1990), Health Authorities are now undertaking work on equipment and facility inventories (capital asset registers) for the purpose of capital charges. Physiotherapy Managers will be involved in this process, which will result in capital charges.

(g) Cost of materials and consumables

The cost of materials and consumables of many sorts will be available to Physiotherapy Managers. Most Health Authorities have a mechanism by which requisitioning officers receive computer print-outs about the cost of the materials and services they have purchased. These costs will need to be included in the pricing mechanism.

Further information may also be available to Physiotherapy Managers. This depends upon the physiotherapy information system and also the information systems available within individual employing Authorities.

Information not generally available

Undoubtedly, there is a range of information in respect of some overheads which is not yet available to Physiotherapy Managers. A few examples of these might be:

- the cost of postage and telephone;
- the cost of energy (heat, electricity etc.);
- building maintenance;
- the use of services from other departments, for example, finance, salaries and wages.

Eventually some or all of these may need to be included in the costing and pricing equation.

Is there a method?

During the past few years, a small number of costing exercises have been carried out in a few Districts. One method has been to apportion costs to specialities by the volume of referrals to the physiotherapy service from each speciality. A calculation has then been made to account for the grade-mix and number of staff working in each speciality, and the costs have then been apportioned. Other factors such as the proportion of non-patient contact time and an allowance for staff who do not carry case-loads, together with recognition of the absence factor, have been added into the figures to produce as full a cost profile as possible (a form of speciality costing).

A further method has been proposed by Joyce Williams which incorporates the use of a Physiotherapy Input Unit (PIU). The PIU is based on a basic unit of physiotherapy helper time. Other grades of staff use a multiple of this unit to reflect their skill levels (grading). The PIU therefore carries a cost. This is not a pure time measurement costing system, as the PIU incorporates factors of grade, time and cost. 'PIUs are used to record the physiotherapy inputs which can be directly allocated to a named patient. They do not include the general work of a ward or department on behalf of all patients such as ward round, administration, record-keeping, meetings and staff training etc. All of these will be costed into overheads as will sick leave, study etc., and walking between wards' (Williams 1990).[19]

It would be possible to develop the concept of the PIU further modified by using other information already available to the Physiotherapy Manager which could be costed into the basic unit. This might include the non-contact time, apportionment of costs for staff who do not carry case-loads, and absence costing. Therefore, there may be several different ways of finding a satisfactory PIU or PRIU.

Clearly, there is no simple or 'right' way of costing and pricing physiotherapy services. What does seem certain is that the most effective method will be to develop a satisfactory means of costing on the basis of costs per case rather than by time alone, modalities, procedures, or any other factor which does not reflect the combination of physiotherapy standards, time and grade mix input, case weighting and input of other resources and overheads. This is an area of work which is now, and will for some time, continue to exercise Physiotherapy Managers.

Information systems and resource management embrace a complex set of interrelated topics. This field is rapidly expanding and becoming of greater importance in an increasingly business-minded NHS. Physiotherapy Managers facing the demands of preparing service specifications, business plans and contracts for their services will need to be proactive in the development of relevant information systems and linking mechanisms with RMI projects. Not only is this area of work important in its own right, but it is crucial in the wider context of physiotherapy managerial and clinical autonomy which could be undermined if physiotherapy were totally subsumed into another service. Information is a powerful and important management and clinical tool, and it is therefore vital that Physiotherapy Managers develop the systems they need for physiotherapy use and ownership. These systems must be capable of performing a wide range of functions as well as providing data in a form suitable for analysis and use by Physiotherapy Managers and others.

Chartered Society of Physiotherapy advice

The CSP has published guidance to its members on information systems and resource management in *Principles on Information Systems and Resource Management* (CSP 1990).[20] This advice appears under the headings of:

(a) *Basis of Practice of Physiotherapy*;
(b) *Implications for Information Systems*;
(c) *Resource Management*.

8 Introduction to Computer Language
M.A. Holland

The advent of computers and computer-based information systems has given rise to a terminology all of its own, frequently bewildering to newcomers to the field. In addition to the many newly created terms, numerous common words have taken on new meanings when used in a computer context. The following glossary may, therefore, be helpful to Physiotherapy Managers as a reference.

Alphanumeric—referring to a field or character set which may contain the letters of the alphabet or numbers—or a combination of letters and numbers.

ANSI—American National Standards Institute.

Application package—a program or group of programs designed to perform a specific task selected by the individual user. One might, for example, purchase a spreadsheet package.

Archived file—a file of data not often required by the user which is stored in such a way as not to be immediately available in the main store or listed as a current file. Archived files can be recalled should the need arise. Storing files in this manner can often improve the efficiency of a system.

Arithmetic and logic unit—found in the central processing unit, this unit deals with all operations involving arithmetic or logic.

ASCII—American Standard Code for Information Interchange.

Backing store—storage for large quantities of data separate from the main memory of the computer. The most common backing store media are magnetic disks and magnetic tapes.

Backup—copying of data onto magnetic media in order to provide a facility for recovery in the event of data loss.

Batch processing—processing of data in a batch, but not in real time.

Baud—a rate of data transmission approximately equal to one bit per second. (Important, for example, when sending data to the printer.)

Binary—a system of notation in which only the digits 0 and 1 are used.

Binary code—a code in which all characters are expressed in groups of binary digits.

Bit—a binary digit, i.e. 0 or 1.

Bootstrap or 'bootup'—load the initial software necessary to run programs. Initial startup procedure.

Buffer—a storage area for data in transit.

Byte—a set of bits corresponding to a single character, generally eight.

Cartridge—housing for magnetic tape. Usually used as a backing store.

Central processing unit (CPU)—the unit of a computer system in which all the processing takes place. All program instructions are held in the CPU and all data to be processed must first be loaded into the CPU.

Character code—code in which each character is expressed separately as a set of binary digits.

Character set—all the characters which may be used by a particular computer.

Chip—common word for integrated circuit (generally silicon).

Compatibility—two computers are said to be compatible if the same programs can be run on each without alteration.

Computer—any machine which will accept data, process it in a specified way and supply the results as information.

CPU—Central Processing Unit.

Crash—a system failure.

Data—facts which, when processed by the computer, provide information.

Database—a file of data drawn from for processing.

Data processing—general term to describe all the operations of a computer.

Data Protection Act—legislation designed to prevent the misuse of personal data held on computer systems.

Debugging—finding and correcting errors which may occur both in hardware and software.

Disk—see **magnetic disk**.

Diskette—see **floppy disk**.

Disk drive—a peripheral unit which stores data on, and retrieves data from, a magnetic disk.

Electronic mail—a facility for storing, forwarding and accessing messages electronically.

Error message—the program will often display an error message when an error has occurred, detailing the nature of the error.

Field—the place allocated for a particular item of data within a record.

File—a group of related records.

Floppy disk—made of flexible material, usually plastic, which has magnetized particles on its surface onto which the data is set electromagnetically. Also called a diskette.

Font—refers to the different styles and sizes of typeface which any machine capable of printed output is able to produce.

Formatting—preparing a virgin disk for initial use by imposing on it a basic structure suitable for the computer to use.

Fourth generation language—a high-level programming language in which those who are not trained programmers can develop application programs.

Hard copy—information output in printed form as opposed to displayed on a visual display unit (VDU).

Hard disk—rigid magnetic disk, often inside the computer housing. Hard disks generally have much more storage capacity than floppy disks.

Hardware—the physical components making up a computer system (as opposed to software or programs).

High-level language—an application-oriented programming language which is generally readable by people, as opposed to a low-level language oriented to machine code. Examples of high level languages are COBOL, ADA, FORTRAN, and PASCAL.

Icon—a symbol displayed by a program or operating system which often allows the user to use a pointing device such as a mouse to point at the selected icon and thus determine the action of the program.

Immediate access storage—a type of storage in which the data can be accessed without any noticeable delay.

Informatics—a name applied to the science of processing data in order to gain information.

Information—the result of processing facts and organizing them into a more meaningful form.

Information technology—everything involved in the processing of data to produce information.

Initialize—a process ensuring that everything is set to the conditions necessary to run the program. In the case of disks or cartridges, initializing is the same as formatting.

Input—the data supplied to the computer from peripheral devices.

Input device—devices which enter data or programs into the computer's memory, such as keyboards. Input devices provide a means of communication between the computer and the users.

Integrated circuit—a circuit contained on a semiconductor such as silicon, containing transistors and other components which perform logic operations. A computer using integrated circuits is said to be 'third generation'.

Interface—the connection between units, such as the CPU and its peripheral units.

I/O—input–output.

K—1024 bytes.

Key—the data field selected to identify a record.

Keyboard—a device which sends code to the CPU via the depression of keys.

LAN—Local Area Network. A data communication system which links a number of computers within a given area.

Languages—various 'languagues' are used to communicate with the computer. These languages can be on a number of different levels, the lowest of which is called 'machine code'. Languages more closely resembling English are called 'high-level languages' and require a compiler to translate them into a low-level language understood by the computer.

Load—when one loads a program or data it is read into memory.

Low-level language—machine or assembly code.

Macro—an abbreviation for macroinstruction. One instruction which represents a group of instructions.

Magnetic disk—a storage medium whose surfaces are coated with a magnetizable material onto which data is recorded and from which data is retrieved by means of read/write heads.

Mainframe—a large computer generally consisting of a number of free-standing units.

Main memory—internal memory, immediate access store.

Mega- —a million.

Megabyte—a million bytes.

Memory—data storage location which can be accessed by the computer, i.e. main store or backing store.

Merging—the process of combining two sets of records into one.

Microcomputer—a computer based on a single chip, or microprocessor, containing most of the processing circuits for the computer. They were originally intended for single users.

Minicomputer—smaller than a mainframe, larger than a microcomputer. They can run several applications concurrently.

Mnemonic—a group of letters chosen to associate with the item they represent and thus make it easier to remember.

Modem—a device for sending and receiving computer data by means of telephone lines.

Mouse—the movements of a mouse on a flat surface cause the corresponding movement of a cursor on the visual display unit. Choices can thus be made using the mouse instead of the keyboard.

Multi-access system—a system that allows numerous users access to the computer via remote terminals.

Off-line—if a part of the computer system is not under the control of the CPU, it is said to be off-line.

On-line—the parts of a computer system which are under the direct control of the CPU.

Operating system—a program or programs which supervise the running of other programs. The operating system manages the resources of the computer.

Output—results supplied by the computer to an output device, such as a printer, VDU or disk.

Password—a word which, when typed at the keyboard, gives the user access to a predefined selection of information. There are often numerous passwords assigned to a system to allow entry at varying levels of security.

Peripheral unit—a device which can operate under the control of the computer and provide input, output or storage.

Pixel—picture element, a dot from which graphics images are created.

Plotter—plots, or draws, graphs.

Plug compatible—computer equipment and devices which can be directly connected together.

Port—a socket in a computer system into which a peripheral unit may be plugged.

Prestel—British Telecom videotext service.

Print-out—any output from a printer. Data in printed form.

Program—a set of instructions given to the computer.

Program language—any language used for writing computer programs.

Programmer—a person who writes programs.

Programming—the process by which a set of instructions is created to make the computer perform a specific task.

Program specification—a detailed description of the procedures which are required of the computer. The programmer uses a program specification to write a computer program.

Prompt—messages given to the computer operator by the operating system.

Query—a request for specific information to be provided by the computer.

Qwerty—standard typewriter keyboard layout.

RAM—Random Access Memory.

Random access memory—solid state storage into which data can be written and from which data can be read, regardless of the location of the data on the storage medium or in the file.

Read—the process of obtaining data from one type of memory store and transferring it to another.

Read-only memory—storage for permanent information such as program functions. It can be read from, but not written to.

Read/write head—an electromagnetic device used to read from or write to magnetic media, such as magnetic disks or tapes.

Real-time processing—a system in which input data are processed to obtain an immediate result.

Record—a data type containing a group of interrelated data items.

Recording density—generally referred to in terms of the number of bytes which can be stored on a magnetic disk surface.

Remote—a peripheral unit which is operating at a distance from the host computer is said to be remote.

Report generator—the process of obtaining a report which summarizes the information in a file.

ROM—Read-Only Memory.

Save—the process of transferring information, either programs or data, to a floppy disk, magnetic tape or other storage device.

Search—the process of locating a record which satisfies specified search criteria in a file.

Search time—the time required to identify an item in a search.

Silicon chip—see **chip**.

Soft copy—computer output which is displayed on a VDU.

Software—the programs which are used to direct the computer, as opposed to hardware.

Software engineer—a person who designs and writes computer programs.

Software package—see **application package**.

Spooling—a queue of data waiting to be output, generally to the printer.

Spreadsheet—a software package which allows the manipulation of data, generally numbers, in rows and columns.

Systems analyst—responsible for system design. This includes analysing the needs of the user, accessing the most reasonable possibilities for achieving the set goals, designing a new system which makes the best possible use of both hardware and software, and aiding in the implementation of the system.

Terminal—a general purpose I/O device.

Track—the path on a magnetic disk surface onto which data can be recorded.

Unix—a widely adopted operating system developed by Bell Laboratories.

User friendly—a term used to describe computer systems and software which are designed to be simple to use.

User interface—the means of communication between the computer and the person using it.

VDU—Visual Display Unit.

Visual display unit—a display unit comprising a keyboard and a visual display screen.

Winchester disk—a fixed disk in a sealed unit. The original Winchester disk held 30 megabytes of data on 30 tracks.

Word—a basic unit of characters or bits which can be processed in one operation by the computer.

Word processor—a software package which allows the editing of documents and the storage of documents for printing or further editing.

Wrap round—allows data to continue filling the screen of a visual display unit without the need for carriage returns by the operator. When the screen is full, further data to be displayed start again at the top of the screen.

Write—one 'writes' to a disk, in contrast to 'reads from a disk'. The process of transcribing data onto a store.

Write protect—to attach a tab or ring to a storage device which physically prevents any writing to the device from taking place.

9 Quality Assurance
A.E. Hunter

What is quality assurance?

Quality may be precisely defined as degree of excellence, and assurance simply means making sure that the quality expected via the standards set is achieved. The term 'quality assurance', however, almost defies definition as it has become an evolving science with its own Society, the National Association of Quality Assurance (NAQA) and its own practitioners in the art. In the ever-changing environment of health care, it is providing some stability and some comfort to health care professionals as it can be seen as a way of maintaining high-quality patient care.

For many years, physiotherapists have managed without any formalized standards. All professions develop a certain mystique, and part of being a professional is developing a body of knowledge and expertise that is unique to that profession (*see* Chapter 2). The development of physiotherapy practice over the last 10–15 years has resulted in the establishment of specialisms which have increased the mystique.

Quality assurance poses several questions:

- Why do anything?
- What do you do?
- How do you do it?
- Is what you do effective?
- What user involvement is there in your service?

Professions sometimes develop in response to their own needs rather than for patient/client needs. Needs, according to health economists, are always professionally identified. So what influence do the users of the service have on the volume, quality or mode of service delivery? Other people also make demands on physiotherapy, other professional groups, carers, voluntary organizations, public and statutory bodies. Another of the pitfalls of professionalism is the information gap. People can be given information, but do not have sufficient knowledge to convert the information into useful knowledge.

Maxwell (1984)[1] describes six essential components of a quality service:

1 *Appropriateness*: The service or procedure is what the population or individual actually needs. This is different from demand, if demand is taken to mean a willingness on the part of the consumer to pay for the service. Need is professionally identified and it is often wrongly assumed that the consumers perceive the same needs.

2 *Equity*: There is a fair share for the population. As the great majority of physiotherapists work with the under-65s in out-patient and acute services, there is an obvious inequality in service delivery.

3 *Accessibility*: Services are not compromised by undue limits of time or distance. Are physiotherapy services organized to suit the patients or the physiotherapists?

4 *Effectiveness*: The intended benefit is achieved for the individual or the population. This forces us to reflect on outcome measures. How do we know what we do is satisfactory and that goals set with the patients are achieved?

5 *Acceptability*: Services are provided to satisfy the reasonable expectations of the patient, providers and the community.

6 *Efficiency*: Resources are not wasted on one patient or service to the detriment of another.

A comprehensive quality assurance programme will involve several components:

1 standards;
2 audit;
3 consumer satisfaction surveys.

There are three areas to be considered:

1 structure;
2 process;
3 outcome.

By structure, we mean the facilities and the equipment to meet the previously mentioned criteria.

The process could be the process of the organization with regard to patient administration, or the process of assessment, management and treatment of the patient.

The outcome is essential to the local standard-setting process and the whole quality assurance programme.

Normative standards are often at odds with the local situation and resource allocation, which has a direct effect on the quantity of work possible, the facilities and the services available.

A starter kit was published, *Physiotherapy Services: A Basis for Development of Standards* (King's Fund Centre 1987)[2]; this was compiled via the system of peer review. Papers were presented to the peer group, which consisted of representatives of the Association of District and Superintendent Chartered Physiotherapists and the Organization of District Physiotherapists, discussed with them, piloted in the District represented and modified accordingly. This booklet was intended as a starter kit to help people assess quality within an individual service. It covered such areas as communication, attitudes, staff records, the environment, equipment and staff profiles. There was a sample of a patient questionnaire which could be used as part of a consumer satisfaction survey. The greatest difficulty with standards set centrally, albeit via much consultation, is that people seldom feel that such standards identify with them.

Although the use of the document was evaluated, the results were inconclusive. Too little emphasis was placed on the training and education in standard setting as part of the quality assurance programme. The issue of actual physiotherapy practice was also not broached and this perhaps highlights the issue that clinical standards have to be set by the clinicians. As the structure and process are often an integral part of the clinical process, clinicians must be closely involved in the setting of all standards.

Getting started

First of all, examine any procedures, policies, inventories, documentation and retrieval systems relevant to the physiotherapy service which already exist in the District, together with other information collected for both local and national purposes. Then, consider how useful all this information is and how it links into the standard-setting process.

As many staff members as possible should be involved and, if possible, a bottom-up and top-down approach should run concurrently to allow for optimum involvement. The Physiotherapy Managers should discuss with everyone how to proceed. It is usually best to start from a position of strength and begin with the best staffed areas of the service with the most comprehensive documentation and information systems. As the standards will have to be agreed with the appropriate Health Service Managers, they also have to be kept fully informed. The National Standards from the CSP and the various specific interest groups can provide a framework for the local standards. All standards also have to be consistent with local policies and comply with national policies and legislation.

Who does what?

The District Physiotherapy Manager helps form the framework and the 'house' style within which the other staff will work. He/she will, therefore, be responsible for the all-encompassing District standards which have, of necessity, to be broad based, but will also detail all the areas to be covered.

The mission statement

This concisely sets out what ideally is being attempted. It would appear to differ from the objective in that the latter is more measurable and precise. In the beginning, choose to do one or the other until sufficient confidence is gained to attempt both. Everyone should, therefore, start with setting the objectives for his part of the service. It is better to start badly than not at all. Simply write down what is done. Remember, a new language is being learnt so fluency will come with practice. Decide on the sections to be covered. These should include:

- organization and management;
- staffing;
- communication;
- documentation;
- patient care;
- staff development and education;
- policies and procedures;
- facilities and equipment;
- research;
- quality assurance.

It is also important to include a definition of physiotherapy to clarify how broad the professional remit is.

The outcomes

These are difficult for physiotherapists for a variety of reasons. They have to be measurable and show changes in the health status of the patient. In many client groups, there is a multi-professional intervention. It is, therefore, difficult to isolate the effect of the physiotherapy input. One solution to this problem is to consider the outcome from the patient's perspective rather than the therapist's. Some outcome measures are easily identifiable, for example, pain, functional ability, lung function, fitness level.

Different staff groups can concentrate on different areas. Remember the standards should be achievable. An example of the standard for organization and management is: the service is organized and managed to provide optimum patient care within the available resources according to District policies, meeting the needs of the patient/client whilst ensuring the health, wealth and development of the staff.

Criteria are then set for this standard, for example:

1 There are organizational charts showing the lines of responsibility and accountability within each part of the service and between other relevant services.

2 There are written policies on the scope of the service to include:

- for whom the service is available;
- services available;
- treatment available;
- referral procedures;
- discharge procedures;
- hours of work;
- locations;
- priorities.

3 Written policies are available on the level of service, including:

- number of staff per speciality by grade;
- minimum caseload of each staff member;
- minimum workload of each staff member;
- staff cover during absence;
- system of prioritizing.

4 The District Physiotherapy Manager and the Physiotherapy Manager (Superintendent) are involved in planning decisions affecting the physiotherapy service.

5 The District Physiotherapy Manager and the Physiotherapy Manager (Superintendent) are involved in the planning process which affects physiotherapy services.

6 The District Physiotherapy Manager holds and manages the budget for the physiotherapy service.

7 The District Physiotherapy Manager and Physiotherapy Managers (Superintendents) are involved in the development and monitoring of the information systems.

8 Written job descriptions and contracts are given to each staff member on appointment, these include:

- job title and grade;
- accountability;
- duties and responsibilities;
- type and frequency of appraisal;
- terms and conditions of service.

9 The departments and each unit of service are organized to allow for efficient and effective patient care within written policies on:

- staff jobs;
- priorities;
- transport.

10 The objectives, organizational chart and job descriptions will be reviewed when a vacancy occurs (or every three years) and revised as necessary.

Each section is specifically written for each part of the service, staff agreeing the criteria with their managers. There will be local differences, and these can be reviewed and agreed by the appropriate peer group. All this is time-consuming and wheels should not be constantly re-invented. Policies can be adapted for each local situation.

The quality assurance programme will indicate how the programme is implemented, monitored and reviewed. As the overall objective is always to improve the quality of patient care, there has to be a mechanism for initiating changes to comply with the standards. It is sensible to stagger the monitoring and review process because of the amount of work involved. Realistic time scales should be used. The commitment and involvement of the physiotherapy staff are crucial for the success of the programme.

Communication

This section should not only cover communication with the patient, but also communication about the patient, communication with the carers and the communication systems within the service, across services, between disciplines, across different districts and with other agencies.

Documentation

This should be clear and accurate not only to facilitate better patient care, but also to satisfy legal requirements. An audit of physiotherapy records should be regularly undertaken to ensure all essential information is being collected. POMRs are now widely used across the country. These records work on the principle of a database being established to provide all relevant information about the patient's condition, from which a problem list is compiled. Goals should then be set—with, or where this is not possible on behalf, of the patient—towards the solution of the problem. Treatment plans are then devised, associated with each goal. Physiotherapists still have difficulty in accepting the concept of contracting goals which are pertinent to the patient. The goal-setting process requires training and there are several approaches which can be employed. The type of record is not, however, as important as the content of the record and the relevance the record has to the patient's outcome.

Staffing

Each service has to be staffed and managed to fulfil its objectives. This section should include recruitment, selection, personnel policies, the appraisal and IPR system, and staff supervision systems. It is necessary to state the numbers of administrative, clerical and helper staff that are needed to support the qualified staff in the running of the service. The knowledge and skills required by each staff member for the efficient running of the service should be clearly identified.

Patient care

In order to ensure optimum patient care, there must be evidence of appointment and waiting-list systems, and the information the patient is given about his condition.

Staff development and education

Staff need the appropriate educational programmes to maintain and augment their knowledge and skills. Criteria have to be set to cover all aspects of development, education and training from the moment the staff member takes up a new job, covering the induction process, continuing education programmes, the policy regarding external education and links with national clinical interest groups. If students attend on clinical placements, then there must be criteria to ensure relevant experience for them, maintaining effective patient care and providing adequate supervision for the students (*see* Chapter 12).

Policies and procedures

Policies and procedures clarify the principles for each service, also the professional boundaries and relate to the objectives of the service the relevant regulations and requirements of the statutory authorities. Policies provide clear directives with regard to referral, discharge and follow-up procedures, and also cover all emergency, health and safety, complaints and security matters. National legislative procedures have to be available to all staff, and there should be clear policies and procedures for therapeutic techniques and interventions.

Facilities and equipment

The standard has to demonstrate that there is sufficient space, facilities and equipment to meet professional and managerial needs. Areas covered include access, reception and treatment areas, equipment, staff facilities, health and safety, and consumer satisfaction surveys.

Consumer satisfaction surveys

An example of a patient questionnaire is given in *Physiotherapy Services: A Basis for Development of Standards*. This questionnaire can be adapted for in-patient and community use, and should be completed anonymously by the patients and users. This is a means of obtaining their opinion of the service and the behaviour of those who provide it. Although there were doubts about the validity of such surveys, they do provide valuable insight into patient services. They can be used as a means of stimulating discussion amongst staff members about patient needs and lead to an increased understanding on the part of the staff about their own behaviour. Surveys should be carried out annually.

Audit

Audit is a system of peer review, an analysis of work and a review by one's colleagues. It is an objective way to improve quality of care, resolve problems and iron out any anomalies in the system.

Physiotherapists assume they know what they do. However, they are often unaware of how other people work, and rarely see what they themselves are doing in a larger professional context. One always assumes that everyone practises in the same way. However, recent case conferences highlight that this is not so.

Audit is an integral part of quality assurance, which is an essential part of the management process. It has not been more widely adopted because people feel nervous and apprehensive about exposing their clinical practices to criticism. It also does involve time and time is often deemed better spent by clinicians 'hands on', as they are notoriously bad record-keepers.

Work attempted to date often shows the information collected and documented to have little relevance to the treatment plan or outcome of the physiotherapy intervention.

How does audit fit into the general spectrum of quality assurance?

Effectiveness is by far the most difficult aspect to examine and measure. Audit goes some way towards this with a systematic peer review of aspects of patient care.

Changing patterns of care and changing practices with professional autonomy require us to be more analytical and evaluative.

In medical audit, when examining outcomes and using death as the indicator, it was found that there were wide discrepancies in avoidable deaths in such conditions as asthma, appendicitis and hernias.

How many people are cured after sports injuries?

How many people regain full independence post-stroke?

It is more difficult to measure specific effectiveness when there are simultaneous interventions, but not impossible. As well as being clinically effective, the best use has to be made of available resources.

The purpose of audit

In times of severe financial restrictions and when under constant pressure from medical practitioners and others to evaluate practice, audit gives physiotherapists the opportunity to show that they do give value for money. This does not mean only in a curative sense, but also in preventing deterioration, promoting health and advising on health education. Audit also facilitates the continuing education process.

A number of approaches can be made to audit. A problem can be identified in a certain area, for example, the length of time it takes from the patient being referred to being seen.

Shaw (1984)[3] lists the essentials of the successful audit:

- the purpose/objective has to be relevant to patient care;
- commitment from the top to allow time and resources;
- participation must be constant with regular attendance at the meetings;
- the method should be non-threatening, interesting and systematic to allow for comparisons over a time period;
- the resources needed should be cheap and simple;
- comparisons should be objective and agreed action plans to implement change should be clarified at the start.

The problem-solving approach

1 Identify the problem.
2 Write down what should be happening in some detail with all the people involved and those who make the relevant decisions.
3 Write down what actually happens.
4 Now compare the two lists.

Change is often more easily accomplished from positions of strength. Pick areas that are nearly the same and have an action plan for these initial small changes. Remember, the people themselves cannot be changed.

Criteria audit

This type of audit is widely practised in Australia, Holland and the United States. Explicit criteria for good practice are centrally set, against which local practices can be judged.

There are seven steps.

1 The choice of subject has to be agreed and should be practical and clinically orientated.
2 Explicit criteria are set, e.g. treatment, management or outcome. The terminology has to be understood by a lay person.
3 An agreed sample of the records is examined by medical records staff.
4 Records at odds with the criteria are examined by the relevant clinicians.
5 The problem is identified by the group. This could be a result of poor documentation, lack of knowledge or poor treatment techniques.
6 Action is taken which may be clinical, educative or managerial.
7 The records are studied again later to see what changes have occurred.

Audit has to become a normal part of physiotherapy practice. Criteria audit is difficult in this country because of poor information systems and low levels of medical records staff. Set simple criteria and as each audit poses another question the criteria can be expanded incrementally.

The process of audit should have immense benefits, both with regard to improving standards of practice and facilitating continuing education programmes.

Further reading

Papers on Quality and Contracts (1990) National Association of Quality Assurance in Health Care, Hereford.

Your Job, Your Safety (1988) Industrial Relations Department, Chartered Society of Physiotherapy.

Health and Safety – Information and Training Manual for Safety Representatives. Chartered Society of Physiotherapy.

Patients Rights (1983) HMSO.

Guidelines of Good Practice (1990) Association of Chartered Physiotherapists in Obstetrics and Gynaecology.

Physiotherapy with Elderly Patients – Guidelines in Good Practice (1985) Association of Chartered Physiotherapists with a Special Interest in Elderly People.

Paediatric Physiotherapy – Guidelines for Good Practice (1990). Association of Paediatric Chartered Physiotherapists.

Policy for the Practice of Acupuncture by Chartered Physiotherapists (1989). Acupuncture Association of Chartered Physiotherapists.

Guidelines of Good Practice (1990). Association of Chartered Physiotherapists in Respiratory Care.

Problem Orientated Medical Records (POMR) – *Guidelines for Therapists* (1988). King's Fund Centre, London.

Heating Standards in Hospitals and other Health Buildings (1978). Hospital Servicing Engineering.

Sim J. (1986) Informed Consent: Ethical Implications for Physiotherapy, *Physiotherapy*, **72**, 12.

10 Management of Staff
B. M. Samuels

In most District physiotherapy services over 80% of the budget will be allocated to staff costs. Staff are not only expensive, but also scarce and valuable. They need to be chosen carefully, trained properly and managed sympathetically.

The current grading structure, while not ideal, offers the opportunity for a physiotherapist to progress through the grades and develop knowledge and skills which build on those gained during pre-registration education. Physiotherapy Managers have a major responsibility to ensure that staff are given the opportunity to develop according to their needs and abilities.

The components of a physiotherapist's role may usefully be considered under four broad headings:

1 clinical practice;
2 research;
3 teaching;
4 management.

The amount of time and level of expertise in these areas varies with grade and may be represented diagrammatically (*see* Figure 10.1 overleaf).

The Staff Physiotherapist

In the early stages of their career, physiotherapists need to develop their clinical skills, consolidate their knowledge of clinical physiotherapy, acquire new knowledge through basic research and begin to understand their role as a teacher, not only to their patients, but to other staff. Their management role at this stage is small, but important. They must learn to manage their own time, to understand their responsibilities within the organization and to develop communication skills.

Job descriptions for Staff Physiotherapists are similar in most Districts and, although the detail may vary, the main responsibilities should always include the provision of a high standard of patient care, the need to maintain and develop competence by continuing self-development, the requirement to evaluate practice, the necessity of keeping adequate records and statistics, and compliance with all policies and procedures.

During the first 18 months to two years, a physiotherapist needs to work and learn in a variety of clinical situations which provide experience in treating patients with conditions commonly managed by physiotherapists. The usual way to achieve this variety of work experience is the rotation scheme.

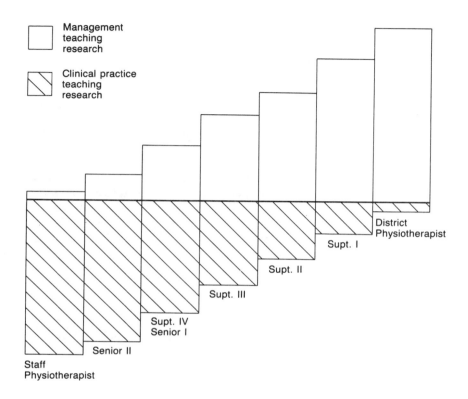

Figure 10.1. The physiotherapists role—time and expertise. Broad representation of the concept

Most District services can provide Staff Physiotherapists with the opportunity to join a scheme where they can work for three- or, more usually, four-month periods. The experience offered will vary according to the District profile, but will commonly include general medicine and surgery, orthopaedics, neurology, rheumatology, care of elderly people and out-patient work. Many Districts will be able to offer a broader range of experience which could include paediatrics, an intensive therapy unit, neurosurgery, cardiothoracic surgery, services for people with learning difficulties and mental illness, and general community services. Many of the more specialized services, or those where supervision is difficult, are more suitable for staff at a later stage in their career.

All rotation schemes are dependent on experienced and competent senior staff to provide adequate supervision, a suitable range of work, a planned teaching programme and, above all, a supportive and encouraging environment.

The Senior Physiotherapist of the section will have set objectives for that particular part of the service and should also have a set of general objectives for Staff Physiotherapists. These might include, for example, the range of conditions that a Staff Physiotherapist would be expected to treat, the standards of treatment required, the contribution to the section education programme and the skills which are expected to be achieved.

When a Staff Physiotherapist is assigned to a new area of work, the Senior or Superintendent should know what kind of experience has already been gained so that they can assist in setting the personal objectives for the individual. All staff should have their performance reviewed on an informal and continuing basis, but a fairly formal review at the halfway stage and at the end of the rotation will give staff the opportunity to discuss their experience and their personal development plan with their supervisor (*see* Chapter 11). The level of supervision required by Staff Physiotherapists will vary, depending on their experience and ability, but Senior and Superintendent Physiotherapists must take responsibility for ensuring that the supervision is appropriate for the individual.

In a hospital physiotherapy department or in many ward situations, there is little difficulty in providing supervision. The Senior Physiotherapist is likely to be working within the same geographical area and is easily accessible. In a large psychiatric hospital, where there may be only one Senior Physiotherapist, or in a domiciliary service in the community, supervision may be so difficult that it is not possible to have Staff Physiotherapists working there.

This kind of situation poses a problem for managers. It is often difficult to recruit to these specialities and this may well be because physiotherapists are not able to gain experience in them early in their careers. The lack of early experience leads staff to choose posts with which they can easily identify so even when recruitment is possible, often at a Senior II level, they will still need training and therefore supervision.

The education programme offered by a District is a major factor in the provision of a high-quality service and is a powerful incentive in the recruitment of Staff Physiotherapists. The education programme and the rotation scheme should be complementary so that the educational objectives set for them can be met by that part of the programme which relates directly to the objectives of a particular clinical area.

Several models of education programmes are available throughout the country, but the principles are similar. Most programmes will involve three elements:

1 specialist education which is directly relevant to the individual rotation placements;
2 general education which is available for a range of physiotherapy staff within a Unit or District;
3 multidisciplinary education.

There is a wide range of courses available nationwide which can be a useful adjunct to in-service education.

There are two essential prerequisites to education for Staff Physiotherapists. The first is a commitment by senior staff, not only in terms of their own contribution, but also in the culture of their section. This often involves their attitude to the clinical workload. It is an unfortunate fact that many physiotherapy services are grossly understaffed for a variety of reasons. It is all too easy for stressed Senior Physiotherapists to forgo the education of their staff in an attempt to cope with the workload. This is the start of a downward spiral: standards fall, staff become dissatisfied and leave, creating an even greater pressure on those left. The situation becomes known and recruitment becomes increasingly difficult. Senior staff in these situations need maximum support from their managers if they are to maintain their education programmes in the face of impossible workloads.

The second essential for a good education programme is access to information. Districts should be able to provide essential books and journals on site, and access to a wider range of literature in the library. Staff should be encouraged to read widely and all staff need to know how to access the information they require, whether this be from the standard textbooks in the department or by undertaking a literature search for a reference in an unusual journal.

The need to encourage Staff Physiotherapists to develop research interests is paramount. Evaluation of practice, which should be a routine part of every physiotherapist's work, may lead to the desire to undertake a specific project. In the early stages of their careers, staff should be encouraged to complete projects which can be presented to their colleagues and subjected to critical analysis by their peer group. With help and encouragement, some staff may then proceed to more formal research.

The development of teaching skills is essential since all physiotherapists in senior grades are expected to undertake some teaching. During their first post-qualification year, staff should be able to prepare and present a session during the in-service education programme of their rotation placements. They must be given adequate time to prepare their work and will need both moral and practical support from their senior. This may take the form of willingness by the senior to help answer any difficult questions, or the purely practical assistance of ensuring the availability of a flip chart or overhead projector.

The staff who enjoy teaching and wish to progress more rapidly should be encouraged to take an active part in any teaching programmes which are within their competence. They might be able to assist with a lifting and handling programme or be involved with the training of physiotherapy helpers.

Some newly qualified physiotherapists look upon management as something which is done by managers, but although common usage defines a manager as a person who has charge of people, the efficiency and effectiveness of a service are largely dependent upon good management by all staff.

A good manager will search for the best way to use resources to meet a set of objectives. The most valuable Staff Physiotherapist will do exactly the same by using the most effective means to help a patient in the shortest possible time.

Much of the learning experience of Staff Physiotherapists in the first two years of their careers is through observation of others. Senior Physiotherapists act as powerful role models to more junior staff and the importance of this aspect of their work is not always appreciated, either by them, or by their managers.

The Senior II Physiotherapist

According to the current Whitley Council Regulations, staff in this grade should be responsible for one other qualified officer or assistant, or working single-handed, or carrying greater responsibility than a Staff Physiotherapist.

Managers would usually expect to appoint a physiotherapist to this grade from 18 months to two years following qualification.

In most Districts, Senior II positions would normally be rotational posts, indicating their continuing training element. The length of rotation may vary, but is commonly nine months to a year. Physiotherapists who have completed two years of four-monthly rotations should have a good basic grounding of clinical skills and knowledge, and may have identified the clinical fields in which they feel most competent. Some staff, however, will not be at the stage of deciding which areas interest them most, and managers must be sympathetic to the needs of this group and endeavour to allow them the opportunity to move across the conventional boundaries.

The first responsibility of the manager is to provide the staff resources required for the various care groups within the District. Sometimes this may preclude a desirable rotation; however, usually the experience required at a Senior II level can be provided within a District and is related either to patients who have problems which are amenable to physiotherapeutic intervention or to a defined care group. Such groups would include services for patients with respiratory, neurological or musculo-skeletal problems and care groups such as children, the elderly, physically handicapped and mentally ill people, and those with learning difficulties. It is at this stage that many physiotherapists are able to obtain their first real experience of seeing patients in their own homes.

Any District service needs a free flow between its hospital and community elements, and the Senior II Physiotherapist is often the grade which provides the Manager with the ideal opportunity to arrange this by devising rotations which cross hospital/community boundaries. Such rotations could be between hospital elderly and adult community services, or between hospital neurological services and the part of the community service which caters for younger disabled people. Many paediatric and obstetric services can also provide experience in both hospital and community settings.

The management role of the Senior II Physiotherapist may include the responsibility for overseeing another person's work and the review of that individual's performance. This can be quite a daunting prospect which requires help and support from more senior staff. Ideally, the manager should discuss these and other aspects of the role before the individual is interviewed for the Senior II post.

A nine-month rotation should provide an excellent opportunity to develop clinical skills and knowledge in a particular area of physiotherapy. Most Physiotherapy Managers see this post as a crucial stage when the individual should identify the field in which he wishes to specialize.

It is essential that staff at this grade are given encouragement to learn by all available methods. Their in-service training should provide them with a programme which stimulates them to look critically at their own development and to undertake more advanced project work. They should also be improving their teaching skills by taking responsibility for a specific area of teaching, either to their own profession or to another. In a District which has clinical placements for physiotherapy students, Senior II staff can be invaluable in helping to supervise students and assist with their clinical education.

Many of the national post-registration courses available throughout the country provide the opportunity to mix with other people with similar clinical interests, and this can also be achieved by visits to, or exchanges with, staff from similar Units in other Districts.

Most Districts provide a programme of multidisciplinary management courses at all levels. A first-line management course should give Senior II staff a range of skills and also allow them to compare the structure and organization of their own service with that of other health care staff.

As staff progress through this grade, usually for about three years, they may choose to move to another District which can offer a slightly different kind of experience in their chosen field. The manager must be in a position to discuss the individual's career plans, and this is best achieved if performance review has been done well and has identified training needs.

Physiotherapy Managers are often berated by manpower planners for high turnovers of staff; however, most managers would argue strongly that there are very sound reasons for a high turnover in training grades.

Towards their fifth post-qualification year, Senior II Physiotherapists should have made plans for their future Senior I post in a specialized field. They should be confident of their clinical and teaching expertise, have a clear idea where their research interests lie and understand the role of the Senior I as a manager.

Interviewers for Senior I posts will wish to ensure that applicants are not only competent to carry out the responsibilities of the job description, but also have a broad view of the provision of health care, an appreciation of the main issues affecting their profession and the ability to make a substantial contribution to the development of the service.

Managers should ensure that applicants are properly prepared for interviews and should be ready to discuss both successful and unsuccessful interviews with staff.

The Senior I Physiotherapist

This grade is probably one of the most demanding in the profession. When it was first introduced, there was considerable uncertainty as to what constituted 'highly skilled and specialized work beyond that covered in the training syllabus' as defined by the Whitley Council. Differences in interpretation abounded and there was often conflict between District services using different criteria for grading. Over time, these differences have been gradually eroded and most Physiotherapy Managers would regard the Senior I grade as the specialist clinician in charge of a particular section of work within the District service.

The job description should include in the main responsibilities:

- the provision of a high level of clinical expertise in the specialist field;
- management of the staff within the section;
- evaluation of practice;
- research;
- education of students and staff of all disciplines;
- quality monitoring;
- development and planning of the service;
- maintenance of equipment;
- provision of policies and procedures;
- self-development plans.

Staff in the Senior I grade are the lynch pins of the service and it is in this grade that the retention of staff is of paramount importance. A manager with a high turnover of Senior I staff should look carefully at the reasons given for resignation.

When first appointed to a Senior I post, an individual may require a considerable degree of support from the manager. The responsibilities of the post lead to problems with time management and priority setting. Objectives may be set with unrealistic time scales, leading to frustration and stress. The manager must agree the objectives with the individual as soon as possible and must ensure that performance is reviewed informally, but frequently, so that timely help and advice can be given. A Senior I Physiotherapist should be subject to the formal procedure of IPR. The manager must ensure that training in the procedure is given so that the individual is properly prepared and can obtain the maximum benefit from the review process.

During the review, development needs should be identified so that the manager and staff member can make suitable plans to ensure that the needs are met. Typical examples might be management training, specialized education in the clinical field, research methodology or advanced clinical teaching and assessment skills.

Peer group support is essential for specialist staff and if it is not available within the District, arrangements should be made to ensure that it is supplied from elsewhere. Most clinical specialists belong to one of the national clinical interest groups associated with the CSP. These groups usually have regional networks and are an invaluable means of support.

The Senior I grade is the stepping stone to a career in management, education, research, private practice or a Clinical Superintendent post. It is also the grade during which staff often take maternity leave. It is absolutely essential that the profession does not lose these highly trained and valuable staff. Managers must use all means at their disposal to encourage these staff to return to work.

Ancillary staff

Few physiotherapy services can function successfully without the invaluable assistance of physiotherapy helpers, administrative, clerical and other ancillary staff.

Physiotherapy helpers should have job descriptions which state clearly what their duties are, and they require a training programme which will provide them with the competencies needed for their job.

Some physiotherapy helpers have been in their post for many years and provide a continuity which can be very supportive; however, long periods in one post can lead to rather inflexible working practices. Helpers, like other staff, need to work to objectives and to have their performance reviewed and their training needs identified.

The development of National Vocational Qualifications will ensure formal acknowledgement of helpers' skills and provide a national framework of standards of competence.

Administrative and clerical staff are a vital part of the service. Valuable professional time should not be taken up with clerical duties and managers themselves should not be expected to cope without adequate secretarial help. Clerical staff need detailed job descriptions, performance review and opportunities for development in the same way as other members of the team.

They also require clear lines of communication and guidance on setting priorities, especially if they work for a group of people or for staff from more than one discipline.

Physiotherapy Managers may also be responsible on a day-to-day basis for other ancillary employees, such as porters. Although these staff will be accountable to other managers, the Physiotherapy Manager must be prepared to cope with the routine matters which affect the efficient provision of the physiotherapy service. Some parts of the service may have staff who are permanently based with the physiotherapy department. These people form an important part of the team and often feel an equal, or greater, allegiance to the physiotherapy service than to their peers.

In conclusion, the Physiotherapy Manager has responsibility for a group of people with varying roles and abilities. All of them are important and all are worthy of as much individual support as possible. Many of the staff will have skills, knowledge and ideas which can be of benefit to the whole service. They should be encouraged to share these and in return should be given the support and encouragement they need to enable them to perform effectively and with the maximum possible job satisfaction.

11 Service Objectives and Individual Performance Review
R.J. Jones

The publication of *Individual Performance Review* (PM(86)10), made IPR obligatory for all General Managers in the NHS. This memorandum also stated that it was the intention of the NHS Management Board to apply IPR to 'most senior managers and in due course to other staff with management responsibilities' (DHSS 1986).[1]

The philosophy of IPR is that people work more effectively if they know clearly what is expected of them and receive regular appraisal of their performance. The key elements of IPR are:

- Job clarification—what is the purpose of the job?
- Agreeing objectives
- What help is needed to achieve success with objectives?
- Monitoring progress—how and whether objectives are being met and modifying as necessary
- Major review and appraisal—what was the outcome of the previous 12 months' objectives?

The cycle then restarts for the next 12 months.

The IPR process

The IPR process involves the DGM agreeing a set of objectives for himself with the DHA chairman. These objectives are also agreed with the RHA and are consistent with RHA policy. UGMs then agree objectives for themselves with the DGM, which are consistent with the DGM's own objectives and DHA policy. In the case of District services, such as physiotherapy, the District Head of Service or most senior Superintendent will agree objectives for him/herself (and the service) with the Manager to whom he/she is accountable.

Agreeing a small number (usually not more than 10) key quantifiable and well-defined objectives is of vital importance to the success of the scheme. The objectives are agreed at a meeting between the individual and his/her manager, and are written down for use throughout the year. Progress is monitored throughout the year, both formally and informally, and any necessary adjustments to the objectives are made and support and counselling undertaken. At the end of the cycle, a major review of progress is carried out (*see* Figure 11.1). The appraisee's manager—in terms of IPR— is known as 'the parent', while generally, the manager's manager will act as 'grandparent'. The role of the 'grandparent' is to oversee the process, making sure that it happens, being available to the individual as an alternative source of counselling when necessary, ensuring fairness of performance assessment and equity of IPR application across a wide span of control.

The Physiotherapy Manager, having agreed objectives with the 'parent', then starts the process of objective setting with the Superintendent Physiotherapists accountable to him/her. This includes the agreement of objectives in several areas, for example, managerial and organizational; clinical; service evaluation; personal development and identification of training (*see also* Chapter 10). The Superintendent Physiotherapists will then agree objectives with their Senior Physiotherapists and the District Physiotherapist will act as the 'grandparent'. The IPR process is carried out at all levels of the physiotherapy grading structure, including helpers and clerical staff whose 'parents' will generally be Senior Is and more Senior Physiotherapy Managers, respectively (*see* Figure 11.2).

The whole process of IPR ensures that the service has common direction. Important service improvements can be achieved to a given time-scale and individuals developed to full potential.

Difficulties may occasionally arise in the operation of IPR between General Managers and Senior Physiotherapy Managers due to the clinical role of the latter. Although service and personal objectives can be identified and agreed, there may be problems for the General Manager in making a meaningful appraisal on some clinical matters at the time of major review. This area might become more difficult if Performance Related Pay (PRP) is to be introduced at the level of District Physiotherapist and below. The PRP scheme is set out in *General Managers—Arrangements for the Introduction of Performance Related Pay* PM(86)11 (DHSS 1986).[2]

Superintendent Physiotherapists are generally involved in clinical work for a significant proportion of working time and, therefore, it is most appropriate that their IPR be undertaken by a Senior Manager with the necessary in-depth clinical background and knowledge.

Recording objectives and review

There are a wide variety of printed forms available for recording IPR details such as objectives, monitoring and major review. These forms are generally obtainable from personnel departments. However, some managers may prefer to use letters setting out the agreed objectives; there is no one correct method. It is important that IPR is carefully and thoroughly carried out,

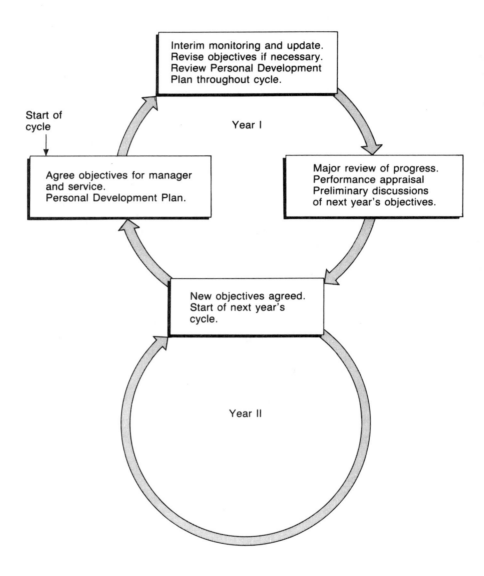

Figure 11.1.   The IPR cycle

setting aside enough time for uninterrupted and private interviews at each stage.

Examples of letters recording agreed objectives for Superintendent, Senior and Staff Physiotherapists are set out overleaf as guidelines to this method.

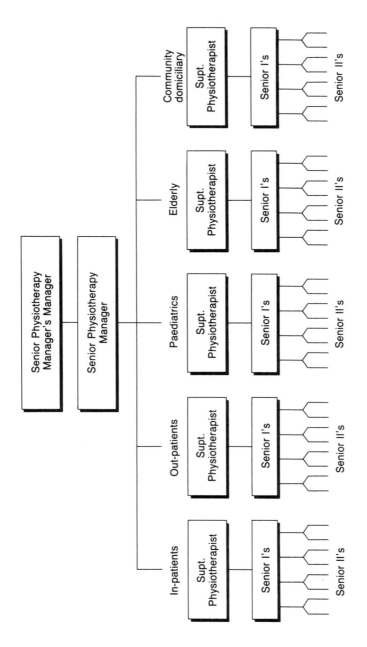

Staff physiotherapists, helpers and clerical staff are also included in the process. The cycle may be shorter than one year for more junior grades of staff e.g. four months for a Staff Physiotherapist to coincide with rotations.

Figure 11.2.   Model of the IPR process in physiotherapy

Guidelines for IPR letters

Example 1—Superintendent Physiotherapist

Dear . . . . . .

Re: Your Objectives 1990/91

Further to our recent meeting, I am pleased to confirm the objectives we agreed for you for the current year. These are as follows:

1. *In-service Training*—to organize a programme of in-service training for Staff Physiotherapists and Senior IIs on a weekly basis for the academic year commencing September 1990. This programme to be agreed by myself and ready for distribution by 1 August 1990.

2. *Development of Clinical Services*—to establish an amputee clinic in the District General Hospital with input from the Disablement Services Centre. The aim will be to improve amputee rehabilitation for the local population. It will be necessary to liaise closely with the departments of surgery and orthopaedics within the Unit. As agreed you will prepare a progress report by 1 January 1991.

3. *Outcome Measures*—to start work in conjunction with myself and other senior staff on developing a system of outcome measures for the physiotherapy out-patient department in your Unit. Various systems will be piloted throughout the year commencing as soon as possible with the aim of drawing some conclusions one year from now.

4. *Newcomers' Handbook*—to update the department newcomers' handbook ready for use during the summer of 1991.

5. *Hydrotherapy Policy*—to produce a draft Hydrotherapy Policy for use in the new hydrotherapy department which is to be brought into use during the spring of 1991.

6. *Income Generation*—to consider possibilities for income generation in your Unit putting forward some proposals in November 1990. To assist in the introduction of agreed income generation projects.

7 *Personal*— (i) to undertake training in the use of acupuncture for the relief of pain. To attend relevant validated training courses and to work in close co-operation with the Unit Pain Clinic;
  (ii) to attend the course on 'Use of Computers in the National Health Service' at the Regional Training Centre in May 1991;
  (iii) to attend the locally organized short course on basic counselling skills during the forthcoming year.

I note your many on-going projects and also take this opportunity of thanking you for your help and support throughout the year.

I confirm that we have agreed to meet again in order to review progress on 12 November 1990 and I will, of course, be very pleased to discuss progress with you at other times as necessary.

Yours sincerely,

District Physiotherapy Manager

Example 2—Senior I Domiciliary Physiotherapist

Dear . . . . . .

Re: Your Objectives 1990/91

Further to our recent meeting, I am pleased to confirm the objectives we agreed for you for the current year which are as follows:

1. *Local Services*—to introduce yourself to and have a working knowledge of the local services in your area. For example, Red Cross, Stroke Clubs, Day Centres, Groups and Associations for patients. This exercise should be completed by the end of November 1990.

2. *People with Learning Difficulties*—to produce a report on your involvement in the care of people with special needs (mentally handicapped) in your area. The report should include information on patients transferred into community accommodation from the run-down of . . . Mental Handicap Hospital. Information must include details about age, diagnoses, where seen and your involvement in the care programme. This report must be available by the end of March 1991.

3. *In-service Training for Junior Staff*—to participate in the community domiciliary physiotherapy module of the in-service education and training programme for junior physiotherapy staff. This module will take place in May 1991.

4. *Outcome Measures*—to join the Community Domiciliary Physiotherapists Working Group on 'outcome measures related to the problem orientated medical records system'. This to take effect immediately.

5. *New Base*—to liaise with the manager of the new community centre in your area. To establish this as your new base by the end of October 1990.

6. *New GP*—to meet the new GP in your area to discuss referral procedures and criteria during September 1990.

7. *Personal*— (i) to update your clinical skills in neurology (Bobath Normal Movement Course) October 1990;
   (ii) to improve your time-management skills and attend the course to be held locally in the spring of 1991.

I have noted that we shall meet again on 12 December 1990 at 10 a.m. but please do not hesitate to contact me in the meantime if you should need to discuss progress or difficulties.

Best wishes.

Yours sincerely,

Superintendent Domiciliary Physiotherapist

Example 3—Senior II Physiotherapist (nine-monthly rotation)

Dear . . . . . .

Re: Your Objectives 1990/91

Further to our recent meeting, I am pleased to confirm the objectives we agreed for the nine-month period commencing June 1990 which are as follows:

1. To review/re-write the handouts given to patients, including those used in orthopaedic out-patients and fracture clinics, by March 1991.

2. To introduce a ward teaching programme in:

   (a) The correct application and use of the continuous passive mobilizer by August 1990.
   (b) Correct lifting procedures by October 1990.

3. To produce a chart for the use of physiotherapy helpers on the orthopaedic wards, showing individual patients and the procedures to be carried out, by January 1991.

4. To participate in the working group on the development of outcome measures. The next meeting of this group will take place during July 1990.

5. *Personal*—(a) to attend a clinical supervisor's/educator's course to be organized by the Regional Health Authority Training Centre early in 1991;
   (b) to attend a role development course for Senior Physiotherapists during the autumn of 1990.

I look forward to our review of your progress on 8 September 1990 but should you wish to discuss progress at any time in the interim, please do not hesitate to let me know.

Best wishes.

Yours sincerely,

Superintendent Physiotherapist

Example 4—Staff Physiotherapist (four-monthly rotation) ITU and Surgical Rotation

Dear . . . . . .

Re: Your Objectives for the ITU, Surgical Rotation

As agreed at our recent meeting, by the end of this rotation you should have achieved the following objectives:

1. To know the indications and contraindications to chest treatments, including suction and be able to apply this knowledge to the treatment of each individual patient.

2. To be familiar with the common surgical procedures carried out in this hospital and their pre- and post-operative regimens.

3. To learn the basic physiological parameters and to understand the variations from normal and their significance.

4. To learn about the drugs used in the intensive care unit and surgical wards, their effects and side-effects.

5. To know the main types of ventilators used in this hospital and to be aware of their uses and controls.

6. To know the common causes, sites and techniques of amputation. To learn about the rehabilitation of amputees and be able to apply your knowledge and skills in care programmes.

7. To interact and communicate with other staff in a multi-disciplinary team, including other physiotherapists, doctors, sisters, nurses, occupational therapists and others. To learn from other disciplines and to be prepared to teach and explain the role of the physiotherapist.

8. To attend and contribute to ward rounds and case conferences as appropriate to gain a full clinical and social picture of your patients.

9. To attend the forthcoming course on physiotherapy in the on-call situation.

As we agreed, progress will be monitored on a monthly basis. However, I will be available for informal discussions as necessary and please do not hesitate to ask for further help.

Yours sincerely,

Senior I Physiotherapist, ITU and Surgical Wards

12 Management of Students in Physiotherapy Services
M. Pauling

The role of the Physiotherapy Manager is to act as an enabler for senior staff, identify training needs, liaise with Schools of Physiotherapy and to identify the conditions needed to fulfil a clinical placement in a department.

Definition of role

The use of the word Supervisor is sometimes interpreted as watching over or directing the work of staff. However, in reality it is much more than this. Physiotherapists who undertake this task are required to have a range of skills and abilities which include organizing people and their patient caseload/casemix, as well as the planning and scheduling of clinical work appropriate to the student's level of ability. It is also necessary to set objectives for the placement which are congruent with those of the course and the physiotherapy service. The supervising clinician must be able to motivate and communicate effectively with the student, particularly when managing their performance. This requires the skill and knowledge to analyse and measure performance, appraise and interpret behaviour. To undertake this role, Clinical Supervisors need appropriate support from the Physiotherapy Manager and staff of the School of Physiotherapy. The role necessitates investment of authority, which goes with the responsibility of the work. Adequate training is essential and other identifiable skills include ability to give feedback, identification of adult learning styles (including their own), developing an understanding of their role in relation to the school tutor, assertiveness and presentation skills, and the ability to set objectives and standards of performance.

We all have many different roles in life and gaining some understanding of these roles gives a framework for understanding behaviour. Why individuals experience stress and conflict, and how misunderstandings may occur. Factors which may influence an individual's performance are personality, skills, attributes and his/her environment.

The expectations of those with whom you interact define your role (Handy 1981).[1] Role ambiguity may occur sometimes because of uncertainty about the role, either by others or by the individual. Job descriptions do help to define this role, but do not eliminate ambiguity. The diagram in Figure 12.1 demonstrates the complexity of roles.

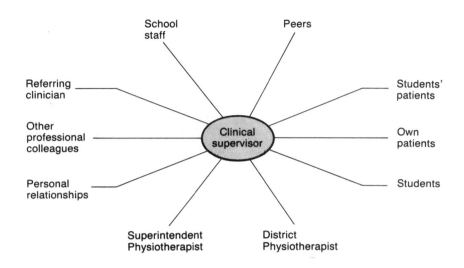

School
staff

Peers

Referring
clinician

Students'
patients

Other
professional
colleagues

Clinical
supervisor

Own
patients

Personal
relationships

Students

Superintendent
Physiotherapist

District
Physiotherapist

Figure 12.1.   Role complexity

Additional aspects of role ambiguity include the area of responsibility and how performance is measured. This is particularly relevant in relation to student performance and standard setting. This issue will be explored later. Another dimension of role ambiguity is incompatibility, which may occur when there is conflict regarding others' expectations of the supervisor's role and their own concept of the role. An example of this could be in clinical teaching where the clinician may perceive this task as the role of the school tutor, whilst the school understands this to be part of the clinician's role. A further dimension of role ambiguity is stress, which may occur as a result of work overload—when there are multiple and diverse roles—and conflict. Stress can be a positive factor which will enhance performance; however, role ambiguity may induce such levels of stress that the performance of the Clinical Supervisor deteriorates. This includes responsibility for the work of others, requiring the reconciliation of overlapping or conflicting objectives amongst students, the school and oneself. Stress management is not discussed here, but before moving to the next section it is important briefly to mention role interactions and the halo effect; that is if you wish your student to be responsible they will be, alternatively those you consider to be incompetent will tend to be incompetent. It is a self-fulfilling prophecy (Handy 1981).[2] Although role theory is better at explaining situations than predicting them, an explanation can lead to an understanding of roles and increased tolerance. Roles and the perception of them underlie all interactions between individuals.

One of the factors which influence our behaviour is power. The sources of power are derived from the control of information, knowledge, interpersonal skills, expertise and status or position. Few clinical physiotherapists at supervisory level appear to recognize the role of power in relationships. Power stems largely from the ownership of valued resources, but to be effective the individual has to control those resources and the recipient desire them. Clinical Supervisors have this power in their ability to pass or fail students in clinical placements. They also possess 'expert' power which is invested in them because of their clinical expertise. This type of expertise is desirable and socially acceptable. As most Clinical Supervisors are Senior I Physiotherapists, they have power which is legitimate as a result of their position in the organization. Some individuals possess personal power which resides in their person and personality. There are several ways of using power, including persuasion and negotiation. However, power can be negative when used illegitimately and has an ability to be obstructive and destructive. Clinicians who manage students need to be aware of these issues and use their role and power appropriately.

Appraisal

It is important for Clinical Supervisors to understand why it is necessary to appraise students in an appropriate way. To accomplish this, the supervisor must identify the purpose of the process, which is to assess the current level of student performance. As there has been an increasing emphasis on achieving results in the NHS, so there has been a tendency to set objectives with individuals which ensure the achievement of the overall objectives of the organization. This method has some disadvantages for the Supervisor because it creates difficulties in measuring performance on a rating scale, which is generally still used by Schools of Physiotherapy. This rating system is necessary in some form to establish the student's level of clinical competence. Objective setting creates specific problems because not all performance, especially a student's performance, can be measured in terms of objectives set. Therefore, problems arise for Supervisors when attempting to rate the performance of students, because the systems or schemes used are attempting to fulfil conflicting objectives. For this reason, it is more appropriate to develop a rating system which will be more objective and this is discussed later under developing competencies.

Feedback

Giving feedback is an essential element of the Clinical Supervisor's role. This may occur either formally or informally, but to be effective it needs to be specific and immediate, and given in a constructive way it enhances the personal growth of the student. Feedback can also be destructive and demoralizing for the student if the Supervisor fails to recognize the needs of the student. When giving feedback, it should be based on observation rather than interpretation, that is, observed behaviour. Feedback is often directed towards the negative aspects of performance; however, the student will respond better to positive reactions. When offering feedback, it is essential for the Supervisor to take responsibility and, therefore, it should begin with 'I . . .' not 'you are . . .'. It is important always to relate feedback to specific items of behaviour. Ensure that the student's personal limits are observed, otherwise he or she may become defensive and withdrawn.

Feedback should be given when appropriate and the crucial questions to consider are:

- when (is this the right time?);
- where (is this the right place?);
- who (am I the right person?); and
- how (how can I do it most effectively?).

Appraisal and feedback skills are two areas where Clinical Supervisors have definite training needs. The types of skills which are required for effective interviewing include knowledge of good and bad questions, and effective listening. Performance in these areas can be improved through specific training courses, including role play.

Guidelines for clinical placements

Guidelines for clinical placements were developed by a working group in the South East Thames Regional Health Authority (SETRHA 1989).[3] The group comprised Physiotherapy Managers, clinicians and physiotherapy school teaching staff. The basis of this work was that placements must meet the objectives set for the training course. Managers and clinicians must recognize that students should be supernumerary. The CSP requires that students receive a minimum of 1,000 clinical education hours and details the range of clinical experience. Consequently, when agreeing to a placement, a manager is undertaking to provide a specific number of hours of clinical practice. Failure to meet such an agreement may jeopardize the education of a student and future clinical placements. The departmental and clinical supervisory requirements agreed by the working party follow.

Departmental and clinical supervisory requirements

A physiotherapy department which wishes to be included in the provision of clinical placements must have appropriate apparatus, including modern electrical equipment. Some study facilities must be available, with access to a medical or physiotherapy department library. The student should be accepted as part of the physiotherapy staff and integrated into the department. General criteria were identified for Clinical Supervisors, following detailed discussion about each specific clinical area.

1 The Clinical Supervisor should be a Senior I Physiotherapist with a minimum of three—preferably five—years' experience since qualification, including at least one year's experience in a particular clinical specialty.
2 Clinical Supervisors should demonstrate appropriate and relevant postgraduate training with relevant clinical skills. Supervisors should also be members of an appropriate clinical interest group.
3 Within six months of appointment, Clinical Supervisors should have undertaken a Clinical Supervisor's/Educator's course. This is a need which managers should identify, recognizing that expert clinical skill and knowledge alone is insufficient to teach, supervise, develop and coach students. The Trent RHA Manpower Planning Report (Trent RHA 1989)[4] identifies an urgent need for appropriate training for Clinical Supervisors.
4 Managers should recognize in the job description the commitment to clinical teaching and supervision.
5 Clinical staff who undertake to supervise students should demonstrate an ability to keep up to date with developments in the appropriate clinical field.

Although these criteria provide a framework, it was recognized that a clinical placement is a matter of negotiation between the school, departmental manager and clinician. Sometimes, a physiotherapist of excellent calibre and experience may be working as a Senior II Physiotherapist or there may exist at this grade a planned specialist rotation, e.g. out-patient/orthopaedic, which may result in an excellent clinical placement for a student.

Measuring performance

Competence

As discussed earlier in this chapter, managing and measuring perfomance is difficult when it is based upon objective setting. Therefore, it is appropriate to evaluate the contribution that using competencies could make to assessing performance. Competency focuses on behaviour, knowledge and skills that are measurable. Competency is described by Loomis (1985)[5] as consisting of knowledge, skills, judgements and attributes. This analysis is confirmed by Caney (1983),[6] who identifies similar areas of performance. Caney discusses the integration of these areas, whilst Loomis looked at the reliability and validity of the evaluation of the competency areas.

Initially, research by Loomis evaluated 86 competencies which were reduced to 55. These were further merged into nine major categories of competency with one area—mangement related to direct patient care—finally eliminated. Consequently, the eight major competency areas were:

1 patient assessment;
2 implementation of treatment;
3 planning treatment programmes;
4 communication with patient/carer;
5 communication with other health care personnel;
6 professional behaviour;
7 professional growth;
8 documentation.

These areas of competency are similar to those identified by Ford (1985)[7] where again eight areas of competence were stated. These included:

1 interpersonal relationships with patients/relatives;
2 assessment;
3 treatment;
4 interpersonal relationships with colleagues/other health care professions;
5 professionalism/ethics;
6 pre-assessment;
7 reassess/update patient records and discharging appropriately.

Evaluation

The descriptive method of reporting observations remains extensively used, despite its liability to observer bias and its imprecision with regard to a student's competence. There are several methods of obtaining information directly from clinical practice, other than observation, including the auditing of clinical records and the use of critical incident techniques. An important aspect of evaluation is student motivation and confidence. This may be impaired by inaccurate evaluations. It is, therefore, vital to evaluate performance against specified performance standards.

Standards

Loomis went on to develop inter-rater reliability (agreement amongst 'preceptors') and the weighting of competencies. It is interesting to note that when the rating scale was reduced from a four-point to a three-point scale, inter-rater reliability increased to 81.7%. However, there remains an element of subjectiveness in measuring the students' performance. In the evaluation, Loomis incorporates a behavioural rating scale which gives a qualitative measure to the students' performance. It consists of four standards. The terms used to describe these standards are 'incompetent', 'minimally competent', 'competent' and 'highly competent'. Several factors as suggested by Levine (1978)[8] hinder the use of rating scales in objective measurement, including poorly designed evaluation tools, the complexity of the behaviour being assessed, the absence of well-developed competencies and the bias of the evaluator. The reliability of subjective rating scales would appear to increase with use (Littlefield *et al.* 1981).[9] Despite the evaluation process never being fully objective, it is important to establish areas of competency and standards which students are expected to achieve. It is arguable that many Clinical Supervisors have such standards against which they measure the students' performance. How else do they pass/fail a student? Unfortunately these are not formally acknowledged, therefore the student remains ignorant about the standard they are expected to achieve on a specific placement. Clinical placements are extremely important as they provide an opportunity for the students to apply their clinical knowledge and skills and their effective skills, e.g. listening, liaising, negotiating and communicating.

Policy and finance

Policy

Government policy has been, and will probably continue to be, to delegate the education of physiotherapists to the regions. This government strategy is in accordance with human resource planning for the Health Service, which is regionally based. However, this has created regional difficulties because of the lack of physiotherapy schools in some regions. It also conflicts with the view of the professional body (CSP) which maintains that training and manpower planning should be managed nationally. The Trent RHA Manpower Planning Report for Physiotherapists also supports central manpower planning. The National Health Service Training Authority (NHSTA) suggests that training requirements should be determined by service needs. Therefore, funding and strategic decision-making relating to the training of physiotherapists must be firmly established in the service. This policy ignores the philosophy of the physiotherapy profession, which encourages its members to gain a variety of skills and knowledge in differing environments.

Finance

The payment of Clinical Supervisor allowances is an area of contention between Service Managers and RHAs. Frequently, District services which have previously not offered clinical placements are unable to consider clinical placements because the resources required for allowances have to be financed from existing service budgets. There is the potential for current clinical placements to be at risk with many regions perceiving that it is in the DHA's interest to provide placements to ensure a future manpower supply. However, unless RHAs incorporate the provision of clinical placements as an objective for DHA Commissioning Authorities, it is difficult to envisage their continuation in a market system. The survival of current and future clinical placements is a contentious issue following the publication of the White Paper *Working for Patients* (DoH 1989).[10]

The complex issues surrounding roles, appraisal and feedback have been described. Some work on guidelines for clinical placements is discussed together with the difficulties in measuring student performance, with some attention to policy and financial problems.

Further reading

Boland, Patterson, J. and Pamkowski, J. Preparing the Consumer of Rehabilitation, Administration, Mangement and Supervision in Pre-service, In-service and Continuing Education Issues. *Journal of Rehabilitation Administration*, November 1988.

Emery, M. J. Effectiveness of the Clinical Instructor—Students' Perspective. *Physical Therapy*, July 1984.

Foster, A. L. and Balley, P. Assessment of Professional Competence: The Clinical Teacher's Responsibility. *Australian Journal of Physiotherapy*, June 1988.

Glace, T. Cadbury's Dictionary of Competence. *Personnel Management*, July 1989.

Greenhall, A. and Hogg, C. Supervisor Training. *Personnel Management Factsheet*, June 1988.

Hogg, C. Performance Appraisal. *Personnel Management Factsheet*, March 1988.

Jacobs, R. Getting the Measure of Management Competence. *Personnel Management*, June 1989.

Manpower Services Commission, *Development of Assessable Standards for National Certification*, 1989.

Mumford, J. and Buley, T. Rewarding Behavioural Skills as Part of Performance, *Personnel Management*, December 1988.

Newman, H. J. Using Feedback and Evaluation Effectively in Clinical Supervision. *Physical Therapy*, March 1985.

13 Managing Research and Evaluation
C.P. Bithell

Introduction

Research is the least developed aspect of the professionalization of physiotherapy in Britain. In the last decade, we have come to realize our deficiency, but other professions, such as clinical psychology and dietetics, began to develop a research-based body of knowledge almost half a century ago. Physiotherapists have much ground to make up and Physiotherapy Managers have a key role to play in promoting and encouraging clinical research and the evaluation of practice.

The word 'research' will be interpreted very broadly. It may, unfortunately, conjure up an image of a large-scale project, which is expensive, difficult and remote from practice. While it may, quite correctly, be any or all of these, research involvement within a District physiotherapy service could encompass a wide range of different activities. Some small-scale studies may be carried out by individual clinicians, addressing questions raised by their own clinical work, or a group of clinical specialists may want to look into some aspect of their practice. For a somewhat larger scale project, it may be more appropriate to consider applying for funding to enable the clinician to become a full-time researcher, or research student. While not everyone within the service may be able to be actively engaged in research they may, through daily contact with researchers, both informally and formally through journal clubs or research presentations, be encouraged to discuss and implement research findings in their own practice.

If we are to survive as a profession, we must all develop an attitude of inquiry, 'our work in both the clinical situation and in the academic institutions must be seen to be based on firm foundations, backed up by both small observational and large research activities. . . . The whole profession needs to become involved. Inquiry is not the prerogative of any one of us.' (Atkinson 1988)[1]

The inspiration and interest of the Physiotherapy Manager is of critical importance in the development and maintenance of such 'research mindedness'. It is likely that out of small beginnings, with appropriate support and encouragement, larger projects involving research funding and full-time commitments will develop.

This chapter is arranged in three parts. Firstly, it asks why Physiotherapy Managers should concern themselves with research and explores some of the reasons why continuing professional development will depend upon their involvement. Secondly, the nature of research in physiotherapy is addressed and an eclectic range of research methodologies is advanced. The final part is an overview of the research process, for those who need basic guidance on this topic, and advice is given on the aspects of the process with which a manager may be involved.

Why should Physiotherapy Managers concern themselves with research?

Pressure to rapidly accelerate the development of research-based practice has never been greater. Changes in the NHS, which are shifting the traditional basis of service delivery towards the purchaser – provider relationship, should encourage us to develop objective measures of the effectiveness of the services we provide. Thus evaluation of physiotherapy practice, which draws on many of the approaches and methods of more fundamental research, may be seen to be clearly the responsibility of the Physiotherapy Service Manager.

Research and the further development of the profession

Each member of a profession has a responsibility to generate new physiotherapy knowledge. A brief reference to the literature of the sociology of professions shows that this responsibility is characteristic of all the members of a true profession. A useful summary of the five attributes of a profession was proposed by Greenwood (1957)[2] (*see also* Chapter 2). These are:

1 systematic theory;
2 authority;
3 community sanction;
4 an ethical code;
5 a culture of professional knowledge, behaviour and ethos.

The systematic establishment of a unique theoretical base is a fundamental difference between a profession and other occupational groups. A much greater proportion of physiotherapists must become actively involved in developing the theory upon which our practical decision-making is based, if we are to continue to develop towards full professional status.

As the principles and practice of physiotherapy have developed through personal observations and accumulated experience (Brook & Parry 1985),[3] this should prove a useful foundation, as observation is the forerunner of more systematic study. However, we should not allow unverified experience to take the place of an adequate rationale for much longer. In order to continue to develop as a profession, and to keep pace with parallel professional development in countries such as Australia or the United States, we must go further and, through systematic research, develop a firm base of valid theory upon which professional practice may safely be based.

It is only relatively recently that research has become accepted as an appropriate activity for physiotherapists, and it is surely not accidental that the belated but increasing awareness of the need for research-based practice occurs at a time of increasing autonomy and freedom in matters of clinical judgement. There is evidence of interest in research among physiotherapists, but knowledge of how to conduct an investigation is not widespread. The extent to which Physiotherapy Managers prioritize and support the aspirations of staff in practical ways, such as arranging courses or supervision, will be a key element in determining whether intentions become reality and projects 'get off the ground'.

The next decade may be a critical period for the development of research-based practice, as the numbers of graduates entering the profession will rise sharply each year as progressively more diploma courses are replaced by degree courses. During this period, the quality of professional leadership and support given by Physiotherapy Managers will determine whether student enthusiasm for clinical research, and the implementation of research findings, becomes an integral part of the new graduates' continuing professional development.

What is research?

Research is close, critical, disciplined inquiry. It is often described as a scientific process, which must follow a systematic sequence, each stage being based upon the findings of earlier stages (Partridge & Barnitt 1986).[4] However, it is important that this is not interpreted too narrowly, to mean only experimental research designs. The essential characteristic of all research is that precise methods are employed and that it involves disciplined inquiry. Scientific method is the characteristic which distinguishes research from mere observation and speculation (Shulman 1981).[5] In evaluating the claims of researchers, we usually find ourselves examining the methods they have used to reach their conclusions. Disciplined inquiry may be carried out through a wide range of research methods, but all have this in common: the methods, evidence and conclusions are available for critical examination.

There are currently two major complementary approaches to research, known respectively as quantitative and qualitative methods. Since the purpose of research is to develop theory in all aspects of this broad-based profession, the best strategy may be to encourage the use of both methodologies, so that the approach best suited to the research problem may be used selectively. However, researchers often restrict their choice to either quantitative or qualitative methods and neglect the advantages of a more eclectic approach. A brief summary of both approaches will be given, together with some indications of what factors influence the choice of methodologies. Such information may help you to judge the appropriateness and value of embryonic research ideas which may come to you for support. Detailed information on research methods and designs is beyond the scope of this chapter, but a selection of books with this information is given in Further reading.

Quantitative methods

The main purpose of quantitative research is to look for relationships between variables, so that causality can be established and accurate prediction made possible. A variable is a measurable characteristic such as joint range or expiratory peak flow rate. The aim is to manipulate the experimental variables, while controlling the extraneous variables that arise from the context of the study. As the effects of the setting have been controlled, the relationships between variables may be generalized to other situations, and predictions about future interactions between identical variables based upon them.

Quantitative researchers first establish what theory exists in the research literature. Hypothesized relationships between variables are proposed, the outcomes predicted and a research proposal is prepared. As the researcher is concerned with replication of findings, measurement instruments are tested for validity and reliability. Data are then collected and the numerical relationships between the variables are established statistically. Various techniques exist for deriving a sample to study which is free from in-built bias. The research design, data collection techniques and methods for analysing the data are described in the research proposal, which then serves as the researcher's guide throughout the various stages of the study. The overall objective of the research is to test the theory deductively by supporting or rejecting the hypotheses.

Quantitative data collection in physiotherapy research employs such methods as physiological measurement instruments to gather data on respiratory function or peripheral blood flow, and instrumentation for measuring joint range, muscle tension or joint loading. Numerical data can also be generated from subjective phenomena, such as pain, by the use of rating scales or structured questionnaires.

Qualitative methods

In qualitative approaches, theory is developed inductively from the data. These methods are particularly useful when the research is concerned with understanding or describing a situation about which little is known. Qualitative research is usually conducted in a natural setting, so that data are collected in context. The focus is on understanding human behaviour from the insider's perspective. All aspects of the phenomenon are explored. No attempt is made to control or manipulate the situation

The researcher is the primary data gathering 'tool', as either observer or participant, and as this is such an integral part of the study, identifying and stating the sources of potential bias and subjectivity in the researcher's own background are essential aspects of the process.

Qualitative research is a process that builds up knowledge inductively over a period of time. The researcher constantly examines the data, seeking patterns and relationships. Hypotheses may be developed out of the data as they emerge, and the researcher will return to the 'field' to collect further data to test these ideas. However, theory generated in this way should not be generalized to other settings, nor does it have predictive value.

These research methods usually generate large quantities of data in the form of transcriptions of interviews and field notes of observation of people and settings, all of which is time-consuming to analyse. These kinds of data are usually harder to manage in terms of analysis and report writing than data which can be handled statistically. The methods employed are generally of three kinds: participant or non-participant observation, interviews and analysis of documentary evidence.

Establishing the reliability and validity of qualitative research requires the use of somewhat different techniques from those employed in quantitative methodologies. Reliability, or the extent to which a study can be replicated, is difficult where circumstances change in natural settings. A unique situation is difficult to reconstruct (Patton 1980).[6] Reliability is established by such methods as checking the extent of the agreement between different observers or data analysts. Peer assessment of data and interpretations by knowledgeable outsiders, perhaps playing the role of 'devil's advocate', may be used to confirm that a researcher has maintained a consistent approach throughout a study. The methods used should be carefully documented so that other researchers can reproduce the original work as closely as possible.

Establishing the validity of qualitative data requires the researcher to demonstrate that the evidence presented is credible. The final report should include verbatim accounts and direct quotations, so that evidence is clearly separated from interpretation and the reader is left to judge the value of the information. It must be clear that the researcher has made efforts to find negative or 'divergent' findings. Triangulation is a process which, by making use of multiple methods of data collection, enables the researcher to establish the validity of his analysis by supporting or rejecting the interpretation emerging from one method of data collection by reference to the results generated from a different method. It is like viewing a situation from several perspectives; the final interpretation then assumes greater credibility.

Selecting a method

The choice of method depends upon the nature of the research question and what is already known about the phenomena to be studied. Using the most appropriate approach for the study will yield the best results. In general, quantitative methods should be used when there is sufficient research-based information already in existence on the topic, such that a conceptual framework may be created and variables identified.

However, when little is known about the topic, quantitative methods are less useful. Creating a quantitative instrument, such as a structured questionnaire, from experience or imagination can lead to meaningless results. It would be far better, in such circumstances, to study the situation qualitatively, to understand the major issues and problems, before embarking upon an attempt to produce measurable or statistically significant results. The following examples illustrate the way that both qualitative and quantitative methods may be used to study different aspects of the same problem.

A Physiotherapy Manager, noticing that many of the patients referred to a Back School did not return after their first attendance, may decide to use qualitative and quantitative methods sequentially to address the problem. He might develop a questionnaire designed to elicit what expectations were not met and what led to patient dissatisfaction. However, if this instrument is based entirely upon his own perceptions of what the problems might be, it could fail to uncover the source of the dissatisfaction. A preliminary qualitative study using observation and interviews should lead him to develop a questionnaire which is well focused, asking relevant questions and from which he could go on to generate numerical data upon which to base action in a convincing way.

In different circumstances, it might be more appropriate to use a mixture of quantitative and qualitative methods simultaneously to address different aspects of the problem and thus strengthen the interpretation of the findings by triangulation. Qualitative methods could be used to explore patients' fears and feelings in a given situation, while quantitative data are gathered on their physiological condition. A study into the effects of cardiac rehabilitation for patients who are recovering from a myocardial infarction might yield more useful results if, while collecting numerical data on the patients' physiological changes and the exercise they have taken, qualitative data were generated about the nature of their fears in relation to their increasing exercise levels.

The overall aim of the study is an important consideration in determining which type of methodology to use. If, in the cardiac rehabilitation study, the aim is to test the effectiveness of a particular regimen, then the quantitative researcher would make theoretical assumptions, use past research on the effectiveness of certain methods and, using an experimental two-group design, measure the effectiveness of the intervention by quantifying differences between the two groups. If, instead, the purpose of the study is to learn about the patients' anxieties in relation to increasing their capacity for exercise, then the researcher might use interviews and observations to gain insight into the factors which contribute to the patients' fears.

The research process

Whatever type of investigation you become involved with, you will need to be familiar with the sequence of stages which make up the research process. The remainder of the chapter is intended for those with no previous experience of research and elaborates those aspects of the research process upon which Physiotherapy Managers are most likely to be asked to advise.

Careful planning and thorough preparation are essential if a worthwhile study is to result and the more obvious pitfalls are to be avoided. The Physiotherapy Manager is most likely to be involved in the planning stages and these aspects of the research process are emphasized. Further information which covers research design and methods of data collection may be found in the Further reading section. This may be useful when actually setting up a project.

For any particular project, the stages will vary depending upon the nature of the investigation. Do not be deterred by the number of stages; not every stage is appropriate for every project. An exhaustive list of the stages in the research process is as follows:

- selecting and developing a research problem;
- reviewing the literature;
- reformulating the research question;
- stating aims and objectives;
- choosing the research design and methods of data collection;
- writing the research proposal;
- applying for funding;
- ethical considerations;
- communicating;
- constructing data collection instruments;
- considering the analysis of data;

- consulting a statistician;
- carrying out a pilot study;
- data collection;
- analysing the results;
- presenting the findings.

The stages which may be of particular interest to managers are described briefly, concentrating on how to proceed and advise, and what pitfalls to avoid. For simplicity, 'the researcher' is addressed directly, as would be the case if you were advising a member of your staff. More complete accounts may be found in Reid & Boore,[7] or Partridge & Barnitt.[8]

Selecting and developing a research problem

Research may start off from an idea, or 'hunch', arising out of the researcher's own clinical practice. Quite often, researchable ideas in clinical practice stem from uncertainties. These may arise out of doubts about the efficacy of treatment procedures, or comments made by colleagues or patients. Research might be inspired by the need to provide information for management. For instance, questions like 'How many physiotherapists do we need to staff a community physiotherapy service?' might stimulate larger questions about community physiotherapy itself.

An important sub-group of research ideas relates to the need to evaluate our practice. Evaluation studies attempt to answer questions about the effectiveness and efficiency of practice. The focus may be upon an individual's case load, or a group of patients within it. On a larger scale, a Unit or service may be evaluated. Evaluation uses the same broad range of methods as research, but it must necessarily be based in the real situation. Depending upon the types of questions asked and outcomes expected, the results may either lead to the formulation of research questions which may test hypotheses in quantitative ways, or they may lead directly to activities to improve the service which has been evaluated.

As the initial stages of the process are undertaken, the general area of research interest is refined into a precise formulation of the question or problem to be investigated.

Reviewing the literature

A literature search will indicate what research has been done and how it has been carried out. It will provide you with a list of references to research papers and books on the chosen topic. A great deal can be learnt from the methods and findings of other researchers, and time will be saved by avoiding problems experienced by others. A literature search should also help to focus the project by putting the study into perspective, in the context of other work done in the area.

The problem which you may well encounter in searching the physio-therapy literature is that you may find very little published work. However, even if you are fairly certain that this will be your fate, do not be tempted to miss out this stage. Your research proposal must include a reference to the literature, even if only to state that 'there is very little relevant literature'.

The essence of a literature search is that it is a systematic way of collecting information. The following points may assist you in carrying out a successful search, but are not intended to be an exhaustive guide. In addition to the recommended books, The CSP provides useful guidelines which are updated regularly (Guideline 10: *Literature Search: what to look for and where to go*).[9] This contains information on libraries and information services, and guides to abstracting and indexing publications and ONLINE databases.

Five steps to a successful literature search

1 Write down your research question and analyse it to find key words. These are words which describe the content of the article. It can be useful to think of a few synonyms. Key words are not always obvious and, if you find a research paper on the same topic, it may be useful to use the same key words. You will need three or four to begin with.
2 If you have a choice of library, use one which holds journals, indexes and abstracts in your area of interest, and where there is a trained librarian to teach you how to use them. In addition to the large libraries in Central London, such as the King's Fund Centre, Science Reference or the Department of Health libraries, many universities and polytechnics where physiotherapy and other health courses are based, will extend their facilities, for reference purposes only, to those not registered as students with them.
3 Ask the librarian to help you to find your way around the library's facilities. Try to be as specific as possible about your requirements. You may be advised to run a computer search on your topic, but to avoid being swamped by irrelevant references, it is advisable to do some manual searching first. This will familiarize you with some of the names of researchers who have published in your field, and you will get to know the subject headings under which relevant papers are indexed. A computer search may still be necessary, but you will find it easier to be specific about your requirements. In many libraries, there will be a charge for this service.

4 It is important to keep complete and accurate records of references. Start a reference system straight away, keeping records of all the details you will need to obtain a copy of the paper or to cite the work in your report. It is very time-consuming to search through piles of paper looking for the article you want to cite, as you write up your research. There are many ways of doing this, but many researchers favour small cards which are easily portable and may be shuffled into order for typing, thus reducing the number of times you will have to write out the full reference.

5 Be ruthless in your literature search. It is very easy to be sidetracked into interesting byways and to move too far from your original question.

Choosing the research design and methods of data collection

Technical details can be found in the many excellent books on research design. Here, some general guidelines are given, which may help you to develop feasible projects and to sound a note of realism when advising would-be researchers.

The research design is simply the plan of activities which will be followed in the investigation. The research methods should be chosen according to the topic to be investigated and the population to be studied, and should be within the budget for the project. Whenever possible, the design and methods should have been tried and tested in previous related research (Partridge & Barnitt 1986).[10] If you are planning to analyse your data statistically, the advice of a medical statistician is invaluable at this stage.

Partridge & Barnitt ask three pertinent questions which you should consider when selecting a research design.

1 Can I cope with this design? Do I have the skills and knowledge necessary for this type of study?
2 Can my research subjects and colleagues cope with this design?
3 Is the design appropriate and ethical?

These questions raise important issues about the feasibility of the project, which it is advisable to resolve before the research proposal is written and before your project is considered by committees who are used to detecting inappropriate or unworkable designs. You may find that you have to resolve practical questions like:

- Is the design feasible in the time I have available?
- Is it likely that there will be enough patients within my inclusion criteria and within the time available?

- Is the procedure I plan to carry out within the tolerance and capacity of everyone involved?
- Is there an unresolved ethical dimension which needs to be considered?
- Are sufficient funds available to cover all foreseeable expenses?

Writing a research proposal

A research proposal, sometimes also called a protocol, is a written research plan which describes in detail the purposes of the research and the investigator's plans. It not only describes the methods to be used, but also the administrative arrangements which will be needed to carry out the research. It provides a researcher with the opportunity to clarify the proposal and ensure that the planning stage has been as precise and comprehensive as possible.

For many researchers, the main reason for writing a research proposal is to obtain funds for the project. However, a research proposal is more than a grant application, although it should contain all the essential information which will be needed for developing the application for funding. The research proposal is designed to help the researcher plan and communicate with all those who must be consulted, or whose permission or co-operation is necessary. It should contain all the information upon which the project's usefulness and feasibility may be assessed.

The research proposal should include information under the following headings:

- title;
- background and problem;
- research questions, objectives or hypotheses;
- literature review;
- research methodology;
- data collection procedures;
- data analysis plans;
- reporting plans;
- resources: staff, facilities, equipment and supplies;
- budget;
- time scale;
- qualifications and experience of the researcher.

Proposals will differ in the amount of detail required, depending, for example, upon the size and scope of the project. However, the type of information which is required remains much the same and you should try to ensure that all categories are covered.

There are a number of points to keep in mind. The introductory section should be interesting and convincing. The written proposal may be used to persuade managers or funding bodies that the research will address a real problem which is worthy of their support. You must present your case logically using data, such as costings or prevalence figures, to show why the subject is important.

Aims, objectives and methods must be specified clearly and precisely. There must be sufficient detail to enable the reader to understand exactly how the study will be carried out. Researchers using a qualitative approach may find it difficult to set down in advance the methods to be used, as these may not be finally decided until some field work has been undertaken. However, the proposal must be specific enough to convince the reader that a particular qualitative method is likely to be the most productive in obtaining the necessary data (Cobb & Hagemaster 1987).[11]

Defining the time scale and resources may be difficult for inexperienced researchers and, where possible, advice should be sought. It is important to be realistic and as specific as possible. In trying to specify how long each stage of the research process will take, you may find it useful to allocate roughly equal amounts of time to the planning phase, the collection of data and writing up the report.

In assessing the financial resources you will require, you should consider the following categories of expenditure:

- salaries and 'on-costs' (researcher and research assistants);
- travel (to set up the project, collaborate, collect data);
- typing (preparation of questionnaires, reports);
- photocopying;
- equipment;
- cost of data analysis (computing costs, etc.);
- postage (especially for a postal survey);
- telephone.

It is important to be realistic in estimating costs and to apply for enough funds to complete the research. For projects which are expected to last for over a year, you should allow for salary increases and inflation. Most research projects take much longer than anticipated.

Finally, care and attention should be given to the presentation of the proposal. A clearly typed proposal, accompanied by a covering letter, will increase your chances of success. It may also be helpful to offer to discuss the project more fully in person and to encourage the evaluator to contact you for further information.

Applying for funding

There are several sources of research funding for which physiotherapists may apply. These include the DoH and RHAs and DHAs, the Research Councils and charitable trusts and foundations. In addition, various fellowships and studentships which aim to support both research and research training are available. Detailed information, including where and how to apply, is available from The Chartered Society of Physiotherapy (Guideline 11: *Sources of Funding and How to Apply*).[12]

NHS funding varies enormously in scale. If you are planning a small project, requiring only a small sum for postage and administration, you should approach your own DHA first. Sometimes there are local sources, such as endowment funds, which may be available.

Regional research committees manage a newly established NHS initiative, the Locally Organized Research Scheme (LORS). This has been set up to encourage NHS staff to undertake evaluation and research locally. Grants are available to 'suitably qualified' NHS employees, and it would appear that well-presented small-scale proposals would be welcomed.

The DoH and, in Scotland the Scottish Home and Health Department, acts as a grant-awarding body through a number of research groups. Mainly large-scale multidisciplinary projects, involving substantial sums of money, are funded. Competition for grants is fierce.

There are several general directories which provide information about charitable funding agencies. A selection can usually be found in most medical libraries. Three titles which it is worth pursuing are:

1 *Directory of Grant-Making Trusts* (1989) published by the Charities Aid Foundation;
2 *Guide to Major Grant-Making Trusts* (1989) published by the Directory of Social Change;
3 *The Association of Medical Research Charities Handbook*.

When applying for funding from a charity you should consider the following questions:

- Which organization is most appropriate for the project?
- What are their particular interests?
- What information will they require?
- Do they have a preferred application format and application form?

As the research interests of the various charities vary considerably, it is important to find out as much as possible about the appropriateness of the one to which you intend to apply. Many offer written guidelines, which you should follow exactly, but others may give little or no guidance. Normally, an informal contact to the administrator of the fund will provide invaluable information about the organization's interests and policies, and will help you to decide whether you should apply.

Ethical considerations

Most research involving human subjects raises ethical issues of some kind. A list of publications which consider this topic in more depth is given in Further reading. This section focuses on the role of the Physiotherapy Manager in assessing the ethical dimensions of a project and ensuring that the appropriate permissions have been obtained.

It is the ultimate responsibility of the researchers to provide assurances that the ethical issues raised by a project based in the manager's department have been satisfactorily addressed. Issues such as patients' informed consent and the preservation of confidentiality might be anticipated. Where subjects will be involved in anything more than the usual treatment procedures, it is likely that the approval of the District Ethical Committee will be required. At the very least, advice from the Chairman of the committee should be sought, and if necessary, a full application to the Ethical Committee pursued.

Each District Ethical Committee will have its own application forms. When completing these, you should avoid jargon as the members of the committee are drawn from a range of professions, including those not specifically related to medicine. The committee will be concerned to protect patients' rights, confidentiality of information and patients' safety. Your application will have more chance of success if you clearly state how you have safeguarded these matters in the design of your study.

Further reading

Research design and methods of data collection

Armstrong, D., Calnan, M. and Grace, J. (1990) *Research Methods for General Practitioners*. Oxford University Press, Oxford.

Currier, D. P. (1990) *Elements of Research in Physical Therapy*. 3rd edn. Williams and Wilkins, Baltimore.

Grady, K. E. and Wallston, B. S. (1988) *Research in Health Care Settings*. Sage Publications, Beverly Hills, CA.

Hakim, C. (1987) *Research Design: Strategies and Choices in the Design Of Social Research*. Unwin Hyman, London.

Hicks, C. M. (1988) *Practical Research Methods for Physiotherapists*. Churchill Livingstone, Edinburgh.

Ottenbacher, K. J. (1986) *Evaluating Clinical Change: Strategies for Occupational and Physical Therapists*. Williams and Wilkins, Baltimore.

Payton, O. D. (1988) *Research: The Validation of Clinical Practice*. 2nd edn. F. A. Davis & Co., Philadelphia.

Ethical considerations

Campell, A. V. (1984) *Moral Dilemmas in Medicine*. Churchill Livingstone, Edinburgh.

Purtilo, R. and Cassell, C. (1981) *Ethical Dimensions in the Health Professions*. Chapter 8. W. B. Saunders & Co., Philadelphia.

Sim, J. (1986) Informed Consent: Ethical Implications for Physiotherapy. *Physiotherapy*, **72**(11), 584–587.

14 Aspects of Industrial Relations
P.H. Gray

NHS industrial relations (IR) can appear complex, but then so is the occupational structure. The NHS is the largest employing organization in the UK and is said to be the third largest in the world (only dwarfed by the Red Army in second place and the Indian National Railway System in first). It employs over one million whole time equivalent (WTE) staff (equal to 1.3 million people, including part-timers). The largest group are 490,000 nurses, midwives and nursing assistants. The rest are employed in every conceivable occupation from gardener to brain surgeon. Physiotherapists form the third largest clinical profession after nurses and doctors.

The NHS is, in fact, the most occupationally complex organization in the UK. No private UK company has anything like this diversity providing a similar range of services. Therefore, NHS managers should not be surprised to find that the NHS industrial relations structures reflect this diversity in the number of unions, Whitley Councils and local bargaining units involved. The fact is that the negotiation of salaries and conditions deals with detail, diversity, conflicting interests and special concerns. It is not a neat and tidy business. For the most part NHS industrial relations has been successful in reaching agreements in the spirit of compromise rather than conflict.

Yet NHS industrial relations, and the Whitley system in particular, seem set for the most radical and uncertain change since their foundation as a result of the Government's reform proposals contained in the *Working for Patients* White Paper published in January 1989. The eventual pattern of the change is unclear and can currently only be predicted rather than reported. The likelihood of a severe shortage of staff in the 1990s makes the outcome even more uncertain. We will be discussing the most likely changes later in this chapter.

The aim of this chapter is to provide managers with a brief but practical guide to some important aspects of NHS/employee relations. This will include an examination of the IR strategy and structures of the employers and the state, the nature and diversity of NHS single-profession or multi-occupational trade unions, how Whitley works and how to discover relevant information, the impact of the Pay Review Bodies, General Managers' pay and individual employment packages, local bargaining in hospitals and Health Authorities, and the impact of statute law on sex or race discrimination, maternity rights, unfair dismissal, and disciplinary or grievance procedures. Finally, we examine the implications for physiotherapists and other PAM professions of the White Paper industrial relation changes through self-governing hospitals, local pay and grading flexibility, local union recognition and industrial conflicts.

NHS employers and the state

NHS national negotiations, through the Whitley Councils, constitute a centralized bargaining system dealing with a wide range of occupations. Yet legally the NHS consists of not one national employer, but of 239 main local employers (Regions, District/Board Health Authorities, SHAs) plus hundreds of GPs employing staff. This number does not include the contractors to the NHS (cleaning, catering and laundry, in particular), or the civil servants in the DoH (including the NHS Management Board) who help to operate it. This diversity of employers within a *national* system whose finances are controlled by government has been and continues to be a source of tension between centralization and decentralization pressures in the NHS. Lord McCarthy characterized it as 'employers who do not pay and paymasters who do not employ' (McCarthy 1976).[1]

The following chart (Figure 14.1) shows the up-to-date structure in terms of IR policy and strategy in England.

The influence of government on NHS IR policy has been dominant since its foundation in 1948. The NHS is almost entirely funded directly from taxation. Health Authorities have very little revenue-raising power (mostly charitable funds and small income-generating schemes). Seventy per cent of the £20 billion of government funding goes on staffing costs. Therefore, it is not surprising that the Government and the Treasury exercised close control over NHS salary costs through either overall control or direct incomes policies in the 1960s and 1970s or via the cash limit each year since 1978. It seems highly unlikely that, even in a decentralized NHS IR system of the future, the Treasury will be willing to give up its control by leaving it to a labour free market.

The government is 'the ghost in the bargaining machinery', always present even if not directly seen. At times, NHS trade unions have reacted by claiming that NHS Whitley Management Sides are a farce. As one union leader told the Social Services Committee, the only person that counted in Whitley negotiations was the civil servant representing the Secretary of State. He knew that the Management Side would not move an inch without his agreement!

NHS IR policy, especially in the last decade, has been politically driven rather than management driven. Policies on value for money, cash limits and competitive tendering, general management and local flexibility are direct results of Government policies rather than employer initiatives.

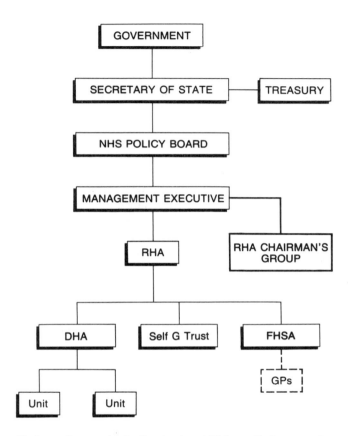

Similar patterns exist for Scotland and Wales, with the exception that the Regional tier does not exist. In Scotland, Health Boards are the main employing authorities.

Figure 14.1. NHS chain of command

The new NHS structure aims to produce a clear and effective line of general management command, running from Units through to Districts, Regions, the NHS Chief Executive and the Secetary of State. In England, the structure consists of the Secretary of State, responsible to Parliament, an NHS Policy Board (chaired by the Secretary of State) responsible for strategic policy-making and setting the direction for development in the service, and a separate Management Executive (chaired by Duncan Nichol, NHS Chief Executive) which will set IR and other objectives for authorities, monitor performance and advise ministers. Similar structures exist for Wales and Scotland, without the Regional tier.

The Secretary of State (and his equivalent in Scotland and Wales) also has the controlling power of patronage. He appoints all the members of the NHS Policy Board, the NHS Management Executive, RHA, DHA and Health Board chairman and members, the FHSAs, the Management Side Chairman and all the Management Side members of the Whitley Councils. That power can be applied to remove individuals who do not 'toe the line' (as was clear from the major changes in DHA Chairmen in 1990) or to appoint political sympathizers.

NHS employers, until very recently, had few IR issues on which they could exercise direct control. They were constrained by the twin pillars of treasury control and the national Whitley Agreements into fairly standard employment arrangements. This was part of the philosophy of the NHS post-1948 as a *national* service with national standards and practices. Employers do control the numbers, types and proportions of staff they would employ within the given financial resources. They could also negotiate local grievance or disciplinary procedures, but few other significant agreements. This frustration at central control has had its effect on the Whitley System and the pressure towards local devolution.

NHS trade unions

Not only is the occupational structure of the NHS complex and diverse, it also has the widest range and some of the strongest professions in the UK. Before the founding of the NHS in 1948, many of the professional organizations, including the CSP, engaged in limited negotiations for pay with health employers. When the national Whitley negotiations for the NHS were established in 1950, both the professions and the traditional trade unions were given seats on the Councils. The result today is the dual system of single-profession trade unions, alongside the multi-occupational trade unions.

There are currently 39 nationally recognized organizations for the NHS. However, this includes nine 'miscellaneous' organizations which are mixed groups of employers' associations (e.g. pharmacy) and pressure groups who have a historic recognition, but play no part in Whitley. There are 30 organizations which are registered and bargain as trade unions; 19 are single-profession (or occupation) trade unions (such as Royal College of Nursing (RCN), British Medical Association (BMA), CSP, and RCM) and

11 are multi-occupational trade unions (such as NUPE, COHSE, NALGO, TGWU, MSF, or GMB). Size varies enormously in both groups, for example, among the professional organizations, the RCN has 280,000 members while the Scottish Association of Nurse Administrators has 350 members. Among the multi-occupational trade unions (most of which belong to the Trades Union Congress (TUC), NUPE claims 300,000 members, while USDAW has a tiny number of dental technicians covered by PT'A' Committee B.

Changes in the late 1960s and early 1970s propelled both the professional organizations and the TUC unions into a radical rethink of their approach and structures of the 1950s. The effect of rising inflation; income policies hitting the public sector hardest; radical upheavals of the 1974 NHS reorganization; legislation giving shop stewards new rights plus individual employment issues—such as unfair dismissal, redundancy and maternity rights—to tackle; some limited local bargaining (on disciplinary procedures, local bonuses for ancillary staff, or new grading systems for nurses and PAMs following the Halsbury report of 1974/5, the rapid growth of union membership and the breakdown of psychological barriers to industrial action in the NHS; all gave both sets of organizations an imperative to change or face the permanent loss of members or influence.

Thus, the CSP (with seats on Whitley since 1950) registered as a certified trade union in 1976, appointed its first stewards in 1976, its first IR officer in 1978, its first health and safety representatives in 1979, and has expanded rapidly in membership and staff ever since. NALGO first became a TUC affiliate in 1965, registered as a trade union in 1975, appointed its first stewards in 1979, but traditionally relies on its network of full-time local officers.

Developments in the 1970s

In the early 1970s, the TUC unions (NALGO and ASTMS in particular) made crucial errors of strategy which meant that an opportunity to weaken the NHS single-profession trade unions was lost. At the beginning of the 1970s, there was a rapid growth of membership for the main TUC unions and a severe drop in membership for the professional organizations, particularly as high inflation ate into the low salaries of professional staff. Members felt that the professional organizations were incapable of adapting to change and lacked the negotiating skills to represent them effectively. Thus, the College of Speech Therapy merged its Union of Speech Therapists with ASTMS in 1974.

However, the large TUC unions made very little effort to actively recruit professionals. It appeared that they did not need to since they were already joining in large numbers. This lack of active recruitment gave organizations like the RCN and the CSP the opportunity to reorganize themselves into more effective trade unions. Yet, the real boost came from the 1974/5 Halsbury Reports into both nurses and the Professions Supplementary to Medicine, which gave the highest single pay awards since the founding of the NHS. The professional organizations were able to claim credit for the evidence to the Halsbury Committee and it proved sufficient to reverse the membership decline. The TUC unions had missed the boat.

Mergers of unions happened and continue to take place. For example, the Guild of Pharmacists merged in 1974 with ASTMS (now MSF); NUGSAT merged with the TGWU; the Society of Remedial Gymnasts merged with the CSP in 1985. Currently, a new spate of mergers seem likely with NALGO, NUPE and COHSE planning to merge to create the largest union in the country; while the Health Visitors Association (the only NHS single-profession union in the TUC) merged with MSF in 1990 following the HVA's near bankruptcy over property deals.

The issue of size, the total number of NHS-recognized organizations and the resources to support bargaining are likely to be prominent during the early 1990s because of the impetus for the devolution of bargaining to a local level as a result of the Government's reforms of the NHS. These will be discussed later.

The Federation of Professional Organizations (FPO)

The FPO (the Federation of Professional Organizations of the PT'A' Whitley Council) is the only formal federation of trade unions in the NHS. Formed in 1980, it is a registered federation of trade unions engaged in bargaining. Its membership currently consists of the CSP, Society of Radiographers, British Association of Occupational Therapists, Society of Chiropodists, British Dietetic Association, Hospital Physicists Association, the Association of Clinical Biochemists and the British Orthoptic Society.

The Federation meets every month, two days prior to the PT'A' Council meetings. It discusses current policies and issues, and agrees on common approaches and voting patterns. It also acts as a mutual aid and support organization, whereby member organizations can develop strategies or gain the support of other FPO organizations. They contribute a levy towards the running costs of the organization holding the PT'A' Staff Side Secretary-ship. The Federation is currently considering closer links between the organizations to deal with local pay bargaining in SGTs.

The CSP as a trade union

The CSP had 24,500 members in 1990 and is the eighth largest NHS trade union. Its membership has continually increased since the decision to organize an effective trade union in 1974. Ninety-six per cent of all NHS physiotherapists are CSP members, very few of whom are also dual members with other trade unions. The Society is, therefore, seen at national and local level to be the effective voice of the third largest clinical profession.

The Society is a registered trade union, a professional organization and an educational body. The different roles of the CSP help to strengthen its influence by giving it a versatile range of arguments to use in promoting the profession. In fact, in the NHS there is no simple division between trade union and professional matters. If a Health Authority decided to cut the physiotherapy staff by half in a particular hospital, while demanding that the same number of patients were treated, that is both a strongly professional issue (about standards of patient care) and a trade union issue (about jobs or workload). Organizations without this dual role may be reduced to ineffective special pleading or driven to industrial action at an early stage.

The IR department of the CSP, with its 15 staff, has four main roles, which overlap with each other. These are, firstly, the national negotiation of salaries and conditions of employment for physiotherapists. The CSP holds the Staff Side Secretaryship of the PAM PT'A' Council, undertakes the pay research and writes most of the evidence for the PRB on behalf of all the PAM PT'A' Staff Side Organizations. Secondly, supporting the 800 CSP stewards and 700 safety representatives and groups of members in local negotiations or disputes. A network of full-time casework officers, covering a number of regions each, also help individual members to resolve their employment grievance/disciplinary issues. Thirdly, the department provides extensive information (through newsletters etc.) for CSP members. It provides a large number of training courses for safety representatives and Regional, District and hospital stewards to try to ensure they have the necessary skills to be effective. Fourthly, the department provides a legal advice and assistance scheme (free to members) on matters arising out of employment (such as injury claims, contracts or unfair dismissal).

Physiotherapists of all clinical, managerial and teaching grades are helped in problems arising out of their employment. Members are assisted in IR matters in every employment setting including the NHS, private hospitals, national charities, industry, sports clubs, prisons, polytechnics and the Civil Service.

Physiotherapy Managers are the biggest users, within the Society, of the CSP IR Casework Officers. Approximately 50% of the officers' time is taken up with representing individual managers in their employment problems (such as disciplinary appeals or their own contracts of employment) or on issues raised by managers which affect both them and the whole profession locally (such as restructuring of physiotherapy management, financial cutback or hospital closures). The rapidly changing nature of the NHS, managers' roles or individual employment contracts within it are likely to increase the need for assistance for managers by the Society. Managers are a vital group for the future of the profession and that is why the CSP IR department devotes such a significant proportion of total staff resources towards helping them.

NHS Whitley Council system

National negotiations in the NHS are conducted through the 11 Whitley Councils or others forms of national joint committees. The most common definition of Whitley is a system of national negotiating machinery, consisting of joint councils made up of employers and unions reflected at District and local level. The impression is sometimes given of an unchanging and monolithic Whitley system. This is far from the case, particularly since the advent of the PAMs and Nurses Review Bodies in 1983, and the introduction of general management grades after 1986. We will examine how far that remains relevant in today's NHS.

Origins of Whitley

The term Whitley is derived from the recommendations of a committee set up in 1917 under the chairmanship of Mr J. H. Whitley, then Speaker of the House of Commons. Its recommendations were aimed mainly at the private sector to reduce widespread industrial conflict. It was taken up mostly in the public sector, notably in the Civil Service, local government and the NHS. The Committee's original views have relevance today. It proposed:

● A system of joint councils at national, District and local level, meeting frequently to discuss industrial relations issues.
● Employers and unions would each be represented at all levels, and neither would be allowed to outvote the other.
● Employers should recognize unions at all levels.
● Agreements should be reached by negotiation.
● Work people should be actively and creatively involved in their workplace, summed up in the famous sentence 'We are convinced, moreover, that a permanent improvement in relations between employers and employed must be founded upon something more than a cash basis' (Clegg & Chester 1957).[2]

The NHS Whitley Councils were established in 1950 with the General Whitley Council and seven functional councils. A major review of the system was undertaken by Lord McCarthy in 1975, but the most substantial changes followed the establishment of the Nurses and PAM Review Body in 1983. The Management Sides of all the councils were reduced from 250 to 50; the management members and chairmen are appointed by the Secretary of State (ending the previous representation system through the regions); and a new briefing system was introduced to connect the Whitley Management members to views in the Health Authorities.

Structure

The original Whitley structure has changed significantly in its method of operation. This is reflected by the fact that in 1989 60% of all NHS staff (580,000 nurses, doctors and PAMs) had their pay determined by the recommendations of the review bodies. This amounted to 67% of the total NHS pay bill, approximately 39% of staff (390,000 taking up 32% of the pay bill) have both pay and conditions determined by Whitley Council agreements. Currently, approximately 1% (9,000 general and senior managers) have their pay unilaterally fixed by the Secretary of State without any negotiation or review body; that number is set to rise by up to 5,000 with a new agreement for Senior Nurse Managers.

This diversity is reflected in the councils. There are now seven (about to be reduced to five) Whitley Councils carrying out negotiations on both pay and conditions of service applicable to their group of staff.

- Administrative and Clerical Staffs Council.
- Ambulance Whitley Council.
- Ancillary Staff.
- Professional and Technical (PT'B') Staff
- Pharmaceutical Staff (about to merge into the Scientific and Professional Council).
- Optical Staff (the smallest—will also merge with Scientific and Professional Council).
- Scientific and Professional Staffs (new council for scientists, clinical psychologists, speech therapists, chaplains, opticians and pharmacists).

There are five negotiation bodies for review body groups which *do not* negotiate pay, but *do* negotiate conditions of service (e.g. grading, on-call systems, hours of work, etc). These are:

- Professions Allied to Medicine and Related Grades (PT'A') Council (PAM (PT'A') Council for short).
- Nursing and Midwifery Staffs Negotiating Council.

- Joint Negotiating Committee for Hospital, Medical and Dental Staff.
- Joint Negotiating Body for Doctors in Community Medicine and the Community.

The Maintenance Staff Management Advisory Panel is an ad hoc mechanism for negotiating pay and conditions for 23,000 NHS maintenance and other craftsmen.

The General Whitley Council (GWC) is the central council which negotiates conditions of service which apply to all or most NHS staff, such as removal expenses, mileage allowances, redundancy agreements, maternity arrangements or equal opportunities agreements.

Composition

The GWC has Staff Side representatives elected from each of the functional councils. (Indeed, the Medical and Dental Whitley Council meets only for that purpose.) The Management Side members are chairmen of functional council management sides (appointed by the Secretary of State) plus senior Civil Servants.

The Staff Side of the functional councils consists of full-time officers and lay representatives from the professional organizations/trade unions. The balance of union seats on the various Whitley Councils has changed very little from those agreed when the NHS was founded. In four councils, the professionals' organizations dominate (i.e. Nurses and Midwives, PAM (PT'A'), Medical/Dental and Optical Councils). The multi-occupation trade unions dominate in the other five (Ancillary, Administration and Clerical, Ambulance, PT'B' and Pharmaceutical), while having membership in a number of the others.

PAM (PT'A') Council

The Professional and Technical 'A' Whitley Council has changed into the PAM (PT'A') Council, with the anticipated move from PT'A' of the staff groups not covered by the review body. These include biochemists, clinical psychologists, speech therapists and hospital chaplains.

The CSP is the largest organization on the PAM (PT'A') Council and holds the largest single number of seats (five). The nine professional organizations in the FPO together hold the majority of seats on the Council (14 out of 22), while the four multi-occupational trade unions (NALGO, NUPE, COHSE and MSF) hold two seats each. The professions, large and small, have the overwhelming majority of the 48,000 PAM staff in membership.

The CSP currently holds the Staff Side Secretaryship and, therefore, acts as the Chief Negotiator for the whole group of staff. The Society also provides all the back-up to these negotiations and the necessary research, for which the organizations pay a seat levy.

How does Whitley work?

We discussed earlier the split of the councils in the GWC, covering all staff for common conditions, and functional councils which negotiate for particular occupational groups. Five councils are full Whitley bodies, negotiating both pay and conditions.

Four negotiating bodies for staff covered by review bodies do not negotiate pay, but they do negotiate the conditions under which payments are made, for example, the Review Body recommends the pay and increments for each physiotherapy grade each year. The PAM (PT'A') Council negotiates the grading definitions which define eligibility for this pay. The same applies to a range of other payments, such as emergency duty or student training allowances.

Proposals for new or amended agreements in the PAM (PT'A') Council may come from either the Staff or the Management Sides. Staff Side claims come from constituent organizations, such as the CSP. They may originate from a local group of members who, for example, wish to seek an umbrella allowance for community physiotherapists. The merits of the proposal may be argued up through the CSP stewards structure, or a proposal of the annual representative conference, or come through the branches, or be a policy proposal from the CSP Committees. It will then be discussed by the Society's IR Committee, which may then make a proposal to the PAM (PT'A') Staff Side. This is often the toughest stage, where agreement has to be reached between the constituent organizations.

If the Staff Side backs the proposal, negotiations will take place with the Management Side. Alternatively, the Management Side may itself make a proposal for another agreement based on pressure from local NHS management, Regional Chairmen, national policy from the Government or the NHS Management Executive.

Conduct of negotiations

Each Whitley Council has a Chairman and Secretary of each side. The Secretaries traditionally undertake most of the negotiations in the full council meeting (except in the Nurses and Midwives where, by tradition, the Staff Side Chairman fulfils the role). Management Side Secretaries are provided by the DoH and are career civil servants (normally Principal rank) who undertake the job for two to three years. This regular turnover provides serious problems of continuity as a new civil servant learns the job.

Staff Side Secretaries have traditionally been provided by one of the major organizations represented on each council, for example, the CSP's Director of Industrial Relations has held the PT'A' Council Secretariat as Chief Negotiator since 1984. The Secretaries of both sides are responsible for circulating council agendas and papers. In the PT'A' Council, the CSP Staff Side Secretariat undertakes all the backing to the negotiations, including the preparation of research and background papers, the extensive evidence to the Review Body, communication with constituent organizations and contacts with government ministers or senior officials on behalf of the Staff Side.

The hypothetical umbrella allowance claim, discussed earlier, may be rejected outright by the Management Side or be discussed further. Thus, the Management Side will need to be convinced that the proposal either has particular advantages for the NHS—for example, that it may help to recruit scarce community physiotherapists—or that their agreement could buy a concession from the Staff Side to reach an agreement of advantage to management. In other Whitley Councils where pay is also negotiated, agreement to claims/proposals may be held up until the annual pay round in April, when an estimate of the cost of a proposal may be included as part of a cash-limited pay package on which agreement is sought. Unfortunately, all too often proposals are rejected at an early stage or are rejected for lack of finance and may only be kept alive by dogged persistence from either side.

The joint councils normally meet every two months, with more frequent meetings during major negotiations. The Staff Side of PT'A' (PAM) Council meets every month. The GWC meets four times per year. Normally, the two sides first meet independently of each other on the same day to consider their own negotiating strategy and tactics before meeting jointly to negotiate. The sides also discuss a number of issues separately (such as NHS reorganizations, GWC policy, or Review Body evidence) which are not raised in joint negotiations.

If the initial meeting does not reach agreement, there may be adjournments on the day or further meetings arranged. The joint Secretaries of the Council meet regularly to try to make progress between meetings or to discuss individual matters or interpretation of existing agreements. Agreement in the Councils is by consensus of both sides. The Staff or Management Sides may take votes on particular issues at their own separate meeting, but there is no voting in the joint meetings. A basic principle of Whitley is that one side cannot outvote the other.

Once agreement is reached, it normally becomes binding on Health Authorities once it is approved by the Secretary of State in England, Scotland and Wales.

Legal position of Whitley agreements

Traditionally, Whitley agreements enabled Health Authorities throughout the country to employ staff on standard conditions. Once the Secretary of State has approved an agreement, it becomes legally binding on the Health Authorities by order of the Secretary of State under the *NHS Remuneration and Conditions of Service Regulations.* This legal power exists under Schedule 5 of the NHS Act 1977 (as amended by Schedule 6 of the 1983 Act).[3] However, it is highly unlikely that any national agreement would be reached by a Management Side without the prior agreement of the senior Civil Servant representing the Secretary of State and the Treasury.

The legal nature of the Whitley agreements is important for Physiotherapy Managers. It means that, unless there is clear discretion built into it, the agreement automatically changes the contracts of employment of NHS staff. This can ultimately be enforced against the Health Authority in the County Court in England and Wales (Court of Session in Scotland) for any money owed to an individual as a result of the agreement. This legal process is very rarely, if ever, used in the NHS, but it provides a legal back-up to the Health Authority appeal process on Whitley agreements.

Communicating agreements

New agreements are sent to Health Authorities as Advance Letters, that is advance notice of changes to the handbook of agreements.

The Staff Side organizations (including the CSP) normally get information on new agreements out to their members very quickly, much more quickly than the NHS mangement structure.

New flexible and enabling agreements

A new feature of national Whitley agreements is the growth of local management discretion or 'flexibility' built into recent agreements. This aims to give local management the right to provide variations in salaries for individual responsibilities or recruitment difficulties. This has been particularly noticeable in grading agreements for administrative and clerical staff, speech therapists and medical laboratory scientific officers (MLSOs). The discretion may take the form of additional increments payable to particular individuals. This discretion is not appealable past the Health Authority (under GWC Section 32), if it is appealable at all. However, it is not being used extensively because of tight financial restrictions on Health Authorities.

Enabling agreements are the latest trend in the process of weakening the power of Whitley agreements to affect Health Authorities. For example, the GWC is negotiating a series of agreements on equal opportunities in the NHS including one on career-breaks. The agreement is advisory, not binding on Health Authorities. It lays down the main features of career break schemes, but it will take 239 separate local agreements (plus those in SGTs) to bring it into practical operation. Previously, a single GWC agreement would have applied to the whole of the NHS. Six other equal opportunity 'enabling' agreements are to follow in 1990.

It is questionable how much local variation there is likely to be in 'career break schemes' compared to the large amount of local management and staff time that will be taken up in 239 local negotiations. Perhaps it will be one of many examples where the current bargaining decentralization ideology overtakes management's common sense about efficiency.

Finding your way through Whitley agreements

There are two separate sets of material agreements covering the pay and conditions of physiotherapists.

PT'A' agreements

These apply to the PAM (PT'A') professions and no other groups, and cover agreements on salary levels and emergency duty payments, how to count staff for grading purposes, acting allowances, and so on.

The 1981 PT'A' Whitley Council *Pay and Conditions of Service Handbook* is very out of date. A new PAM (PT'A') handbook should be issued in 1990. A copy should be available for managers from the personnel department, alternatively, from the local CSP steward. Amendments to the 1981 handbook have been given in Advance Letters and the personnel department should have a complete set.

General Whitley Council Handbook 1984

These agreements apply to all NHS staff, covering travelling expenses, public holidays, redundancy, protection, NHS reorganization, telephone allowances, grievance procedures, appeals on service conditions, and so forth.

The handbook is regularly updated (particularly travelling expenses). Again copies should be available from the personnel department or accessed via the CSP District Steward.

Find your way through the Whitley agreements by using the following:

1 *The index to the handbooks and contents page*: The index is clear in both handbooks. The contents pages of the 1981 PT'A' handbook are very confusing. Be careful not to mix up the agreements for the other 11 professions with those for physiotherapy in the same handbook. By contrast, the GWC contents pages are easy to use.

2 *Advice on interpreting Whitley Agreements*: To be found in the CSP steward handbook, Part 1, available for reference from the CSP steward. This is particularly good on maternity leave and emergency duty agreements. It is to be updated in 1990.

3 *Management circulars*: Some Health Authorities produce special handbooks of procedures for managers which contain advice on agreements. Copies, if they exist, are available from personnel departments.

4 *CSP Stewards News*: This is issued monthly and is available in most physiotherapy departments, containing detailed advice on new agreements.

5 *CSP Journal: IR News Page*: Major items and full information on any new agreements, often in greater detail than in Stewards News.

6 *Health Service Journal or Therapy Weekly*: Both publications contain relevant information on GWC agreements (*Health Service Journal*) or PAM (PT'A') agreements (*Therapy Weekly*).

Pay Review Body

From 1950 until 1982, physiotherapist salaries were negotiated annually in the PT'A' Whitley Council. In the 1950s and much of the 1960s, salaries were comparatively low, but caused little real discontent in a period of low inflation. Physiotherapists' pay had always been collectively negotiated with the other PAMs plus speech therapists. Occasionally, pay was referred to special tribunals or enquiries, which generally resulted in little more than standing still for short periods on low salaries.

The Halsbury Report of 1974/5 was an exception. It awarded increases of 20–35%, but at a time when inflation was running at almost 25% per annum. Afterwards, there was a steady decline in pay because of Government incomes policies and cash limits over the following years. The 1980 Clegg Commission (whose conclusions on hours and professional work of PAM staff caused industrial action for the first time from physiotherapists) was only a temporary improvement before the decline of the following years.

Thus, by 1982, the profession was pushing very hard for a pay mechanism which would improve salaries and prevent this roller-coaster pattern of pay values. The solution came out of the negotiations to end the bitter 1982 NHS pay dispute. This had lasted for nine months and created an unprecedented unified approach from staff, even where groups were not participating in industrial action. The Government clearly decided that it did not wish to face such a united front again. It therefore offered to create a new Pay Review Body (PRB) to cover nurses, midwives, health visitors and PAMs.

The CSP and most of the other PT'A' organizations accepted the offer. The speech therapists, on the advice of their union ASTMS, declined the offer and decided to negotiate alone for the first time. The Prime Minister announced the formation of the Review Body in 1983. Its first reports were produced in April 1984. The Review Body covers both nurses and PAM staff, but under entirely separate references. It receives separate evidence and produces a separate report. A review body for doctors had existed since 1960.

The membership of the PAM Review Body consists of eight people appointed by the Prime Minister. They are mostly distinguished individuals from industry, commerce, universities or retired civil servants. The experience of the PAM Reports since 1984 has been that the PRB has operated fairly and jealously guards its independence.

It operates as a form of third party arbitration. Both the PT'A' Staff Side and the DoH submit evidence to the Review Body, and are subsequently orally questioned on this information. The PAM (PT'A') Staff Side puts a large effort—organized by the CSP—into the production of extensive and technically detailed evidence on vacancy rates, future manpower projections, morale, comparative salary rates, allowances and so on. The Review Body reaches its own conclusion on salary rates, which appear in its reports. It has the advantage over Whitley negotiations because it is not, and has always resisted being, tied to the NHS cash limit for pay. The PRB's duty, laid down in its terms of reference, is to make recommendations to the Prime Minister on the pay it feels is appropriate.

The Prime Minister is committed to accepting the PRB's full reports and salary recommendations 'unless there are obviously compelling reasons for not doing so'. It should be noted that the Government has found such compelling reasons in three out of the seven reports since 1984. In 1985 and 1990, the awards were paid in two instalments, for example, 8% payable from 1 April 1990 with the rest of a 10.2% award payable from 1 January 1991. A previous delay of three months for payment in 1986 led the Review Body to state, 'The Community cannot expect to sustain and improve the quality of health care at the expense of those providing it' (PRB 1987).[4]

Despite these delays, physiotherapists have done far better than before in increasing pay and sustaining the improvements in salary. Real pay—taking inflation into account—for physiotherapists has increased by over 50% between 1974 and 1990.

The Review Body can only make pay recommendations. Conditions have to be negotiated by the PAM (PT'A' Council).

The Review Bodies in 1990, appear to be under threat of potential abolition, following comments in the press by the NHS Director of Personnel, Mr Caines. However, the PAMs, nurses and doctors are all fighting a strong political battle to prevent their removal. It is likely that they will be retained, despite the obvious difficulties they may cause for SGTs who wish to have local pay bargaining.

General Managers and individual employment packages

A new third alternative form of pay determination for the NHS has appeared since 1986—unilateral determination by the Secretary of State. General Managers have been pulled out of collective bargaining by what can be described as 'salame tactics'. In 1986, 700 Unit, District and Regional Managers were pulled out of the Whitley system, put on three-year short-term contracts, with PRP. In 1987, a further 1,200 managers on District Boards and in 1988 7,000 managers accountable to UGMs were added, without the short-term contract. That number could increase by a further 6,000 in 1990 if a new deal for Senior Nurse Managers is negotiated. The eventual aim seems to be to remove a large proportion of managers from collective bargaining and, in effect, to remove recognition of the professional organizations and trade unions.

Some managers, within the salary rates fixed by the Secretary of State, can negotiate their own 'individual employment package'. This is perceived to be a future pattern where staff become fragmented individuals rewarded for their individual contribution. However, its advocates overlook the problems of administering 'individual packages' for up to one million staff, the fact that the rates are largely pre-determined by the Secretary of State and that collective bargaining by staff is more likely to produce better awards than itemized individual bargaining.

Impact of employment law on Physiotherapy Managers

Introduction

This section provides managers with a basic guide to the legal rules and the agreed procedures which affect Physiotherapy Managers or staff. The issues of employment, sex or race discrimination and equal opportunity policies and maternity rights.

The last 25 years have produced a large amount of legislation which directly or indirectly affects the employment status of physiotherapists. The main acts include the Employment Protection (Consolidation) Act 1978 (amended by the 1980 Employment Act), the Sex Discrimination Acts of 1975 and 1986, the Race Relations Act 1965 and the Health & Safety at Work Act 1974.

There are also binding GWC agreements, such as Section 45 on redundancy payments, Section 6 on maternity leave, Section 33 on collective disputes procedures, Section 32 for appeals on the application of Whitley agreements, and Section 39 on the right of staff to be consulted. Finally, at Health Authority or SGT level, it is necessary to be aware of the local agreements on general grievance or disciplinary procedures.

This is a formidable collection of material. However, for most managers it is sufficient to have a general knowledge of the provisions and to know where to find the detailed information when it is needed.

Status of staff

It is important to distinguish between three different terms which are sometimes used interchangeably and confusingly.

- *Employer*: A company, organization, statutory body or individual who pays another person and holds their contract of employment to carry out work under the orders of the paymaster.

  Managers are *not* employers. They are employees who are paid to plan and direct the work of other staff. The only exception would be physiotherapists who both owned and managed a business of their own.
- *Employee*: An individual who is paid to undertake specific work under a contract of service, that is a contract of employment, for an employing organization such as an NHS Health Authority or a private practitioner.
- *Self-employed*: Someone who works as an independent contractor under a contract *for* services. They are paid fees not a salary and have few if any rights under employment legislation.

Discrimination

Most forms of discrimination are unlawful or subject to challenge by employees. Employers cannot legally discriminate against employees or potential employees on the grounds of sex, marriage, race, or union or non-union membership. It is not unlawful, but it is very bad practice—subject to action through grievance procedures—to discriminate on grounds of age, sexual orientation, or religion (N.B. religious discrimination is unlawful in Northern Ireland). However, if an age limit is fixed, for example 30 years or under for a physiotherapist to be considered for a job, this may be *'indirect'* sexual discrimination and, as such, be unlawful. This is because fewer women than men may be eligible for jobs in a particular age group because they have taken time out of employment to have children.

Sex or marriage discrimination

Discrimination in employment means less favourable treatment of a man or a woman on grounds of their sex or because they are married. This applies under the 1975 and 1986 Sex Discrimination Acts. Managers must not discriminate:

- In the original advertising or in the interviews for a post. For example, managers must not ask a woman about how she intends to have her children minded during working hours, nor must they base their judgement of her suitability on that issue; the same question would never be asked of a man.
- In the terms on which the job is offered to an applicant.
- In deciding who is offered the job.
- In opportunities for promotion or training.
- For other benefits to employees.
- In dismissals.
- If someone takes a case against a manager to an Industrial Tribunal for discrimination, it is illegal for the manager to victimize him or her afterwards.
- In pregnancy. A decision to dismiss a pregnant physiotherapist employee is likely to be automatically unfair if the reason or principal reason for the dismissal is that she is pregnant or any other reason connected with pregnancy.
- In retirement age. The 1986 Sex Discrimination Act gives equal right to men and women in the same employment to retire at the same standard age, for example up to 65 years. Pension ages can be different. However, a recent European court case may change this position. The fact that only female physiotherapists can retire and have a pension at the age of 55 while men wait until they are 60 or 65 years old may be challenged under the European Court decision.

Race discrimination

This means treating one person less favourably than another on racial grounds, which includes colour, race, nationality, ethnic or national origin.
  An employer must not discriminate:

- in interviews or advertising for the job;
- in the terms on which the job is offered;
- deciding who is offered the job;
- in opportunities for promotion, transfer or training;
- in benefits to employees;
- in dismissals;

- indirect discrimination can apply if a requirement for a job is made which is not vital to that job and which one racial group would find more difficult to meet than another, for example a refusal to allow the wearing of turbans;
- an employee who takes the manager to an industrial tribunal claiming racial discrimination.

The NHS employs significant numbers of staff from ethnic minorities but does not have any national policy. This is likely to be a subject of increased importance for managers in the 1990s.

Trade union membership or non-membership

The 1978 Employment Protection Act lays down that the employer will be automatically guilty of unfair dismissal if an employee is dismissed for:

- attempting to become a member or becoming a member of an independent trade union;
- taking part in trade union activities at an appropriate time, which is normally outside working hours, or inside working hours with the agreement of the management;
- refusing to become a member of a particular trade union. However, qualification and current state registration of physiotherapists (which may imply CSP membership) is a legal requirement for NHS employment under the NHS Professions Supplementary to Medicine Act.

Employees can also complain to an industrial tribunal if they are penalized short of dismissal or if they are made redundant for any of the above actions, for example, if a shop steward is harassed or discriminated against in promotion, legal action may be brought while the person is still employed. There is also the possibility that the CSP or other trade union would take out a grievance which could not be defended.

Industrial action does not count as union activities and in certain circumstances staff can be dismissed without access to an industrial tribunal. The 1990 Employment Act makes this discrimination worse by permitting the selective dismissal of individual strikers instead of dismissing all strikers together. No other EEC country has such discriminatory laws.

Criminal offences

Certain staff have a legal right to refuse to disclose that they have been convicted of certain criminal offences.

The Rehabilitation of Offenders Act 1974 provides that 'a spent' conviction shall not be a proper ground for dismissing a person from an office, profession, occupation or employment.

However, physiotherapists and other professions supplementary to medicine are exempted from the Act. This means that, if asked on the application form, physiotherapists should reveal any criminal convictions, can be refused employment if the manager considers the conviction relevant, and can be dismissed if the physiotherapist has hidden the conviction and it is relevant. In most cases, serious criminal convictions are automatically reported to the CSP ethical committee and the State Registration Board by the police. The CSP and the CPSM may then decide to strike off or take some other penalty against the individual.

Other staff (such as secretaries, porters and clerks) who may have had sentences of 30 months or less do not have to disclose their convictions after a specified time, which is varied, but is not more than 10 years and not less than six months. A person can lie about this and is legally entitled not to disclose their convictions if employed. If their past is subsequently discovered, such a person cannot be dismissed for this reason.

Legal rights of part-time staff

An employee who works more than 16 hours per week is classified for purposes of the law as a 'full-time' employee. These employees achieve a series of legal rights earlier than part-timers.

Part-time staff are often an important part of the physiotherapy work force, for example, approximately 37% of all NHS physiotherapists work on a part-time basis. The high vacancy rate in physiotherapy (10% in 1989) plus the demographic shortfall of school leavers are likely to make part-time physiotherapists an increasingly important part of the work force. This implies the need to increase facilities for child care, flexible working, job sharing, and so on, to attract and retain such staff.

There are two categories of part-time workers for the purposes of employment legislation:

- staff who work at least eight hours, but less than 16 hours per week;
- staff who work less than eight hours per week.

The staff who work less than eight hours have very few rights under the employment legislation (with the exception of the right not to be discriminated against). They do have the right to maternity leave under Section 6 of the GWC agreements. Employees who work at least eight hours, but less than 16 hours per week, can acquire most of the employment rights, but will have to wait for five years. After five years, they have the legal right:

- not to be dismissed because of pregnancy;
- to get maternity pay;
- to receive time off for ante-natal care;
- to receive an itemized pay statement;

- to receive minimum notice of dismissal;
- to receive a written statement of the reasons for dismissal;
- not to be dismissed unfairly;
- to receive a written statement of the main terms and conditions of employment;
- to receive a redundancy payment, if appropriate, and time off to look for another job.

Maternity rights

NHS employees are covered by the extensive provisions of the NHS Maternity Leave agreement, Section 6 of GWC Handbook. This agreement covers the amount of service needed (one or two years), the amount of leave, the rate of pay, the right to return, the notice period required and the variations of contract.

Right to return

Staff have the right to return to the same job which they left. Difficulties sometimes arise over staff employed as locums during the maternity leave, but it should be made clear that it is the job of the physiotherapist on maternity leave, if she wishes to return.

Return to same employer?

The GWC agreement enables staff to take a post with another NHS employer after maternity leave, and, as long as they work for three months after, there is no loss of maternity pay.

Request to work part time?

A full-time employee does not have the right to demand part-time working on return from maternity leave. She has the right to *ask* and the GWC agreement says 'the request will not be unreasonably refused'. It can be challenged if the refusal is unreasonable (for example 'we don't have part-timers in our department').

Other legal issues are covered in chapter 5.

Further reading

Pay Review Body (1990) Review Body for Nursing Staff, Midwives, Health Visitors, and Professions Allied to Medicine. *Seventh Report on Professions Allied to Medicine 1990.* HMSO, London.

Clegg, H. A. (1979) Standing Commission on Pay and Comparability. *Report No 4: Professions Supplementary to Medicine and Speech Therapy.*

Halsbury (1975) *Report of the Committee of Inquiry into the Pay and Related Conditions of Service of the Professions Supplementary to Medicine and Speech Therapists.* HMSO, London.
HMSO (1989) *Working for Patients.*
Department of Health (1990) Warlow Report.
Social Service Committee (1989) *Resourcing the NHS—Whitley Councils.* 3rd Report 1989.
Trent Region (1989) *IR in Self-Governing Hospitals.*

There is very little up-to-date published information on NHS industrial relations. The most recent study is that in the House of Commons Social Services Committee Report on the Whitley Councils in 1989 (*see* above). It is also useful for its comments on local bargaining.

The best detailed introduction is a 1981 TUC report *Improving Industrial Relations in the NHS.* This gives an excellent analysis of the national bargaining structure. A more recent publication is a 1989 chapter entitled 'Industrial Relations in the NHS since 1979' by R. Mailly, in *IR in the Public Services* by R. Mailly and S. J. Dimmock (1979, Routledge, London).

A recent analysis of general legal issues in the public sector is in G. Morris *Law and the Public Sector* (1990).

More general text books on industrial relations are G. F. Thomason *A Textbook of Industrial Relations Management* (1984, IPM) which is very readable, and a more detailed text is M. Salaman *Industrial Relations—Theory and Practice* (1987, Prentice Hall).

15 Contracts of Employment
P.H. Gray

Introduction

Physiotherapy Managers are often confused and alarmed by the legal and procedural requirements relating to the employment of staff. It is the aim of this chapter to provide managers with a guide to the rules of employment and contracts of employment. It includes information on the legal aspects of who is an employee, paperwork preparation for employing staff, job descriptions, advertising, interviewing staff and the special requirements of state registration. It goes on to consider the contract of employment and changes to contracts, the effect of collective agreements, grievance procedures, and the disciplining of staff. It demonstrates that with reasonable care and fairness, managers can find their way through the legal and other requirements of employing staff without difficulty.

If you run into problems as a manager in the employment of staff, you should first consult your personnel department for advice. If you have problems with your own contract of employment, you can seek advice from the CSP industrial relations department via your steward.

Who is an employee?

There is considerable confusion about who can be classified as an employee and who is self-employed, or what the law calls an independent contractor. The distinction can be very important in terms of taxation and National Insurance liability. It also has a significant effect on the legal rights of individuals under employment legislation.

In the NHS, the vast majority of staff will be employees. Most private practitioners will be self-employed. However, even in the NHS, the situation is becoming more mixed. Management consultants are being employed in large numbers and will frequently be self-employed. Outside contractors under the competitive tendering process, for example for cleaning and catering, will bring their own employees with them. GPs providing the family doctor service for the NHS are almost all self-employed.

The law distinguishes the following:

An employee works under a contract of employment which is a contract of service. It is a voluntary agreement where the work of the employee is clearly under the direct control of the employer. The employee has to undertake the work in person; the employer gives the orders on how and when to work; the employer's tools and equipment are used; the hours, holidays and sick pay arrangements are decided by the employer and equally the employer is responsible for deducting income tax and National Insurance contributions. Most of all, an employee working under a contract of service cannot be said to be in business for himself.

An independent contractor or *self-employed person* would normally pay his own income tax and National Insurance contributions; come to work when he chooses and if he cannot go to work himself he can employ someone else to take his place; he generally has control of how he works from day to day, often having some capital stake at risk in his own business, he corrects unsatisfactory work in his own time and at his own expense, and frequently works for more than one client.

Generally speaking, the legal rights of the self-employed are limited to the particular terms of the contract for services, health and safety and the right not to be discriminated against. Employees, particularly those working more than eight hours per week, are covered both by a wide range of legal requirements and by specific collective agreements negotiated with their employer.

Who is the employer?

Managers are not employers. They are employees acting on behalf of the employers. Employers of physiotherapists are mostly District, Area or Special Health Authorities, SGTs or GP practices. Outside of the NHS, the employer may be a charity, a company, a private hospital or any private practitioner. The employer pays the staff out of the organization's resources. The employer has a legal responsibility in holding the contracts of employment of the staff who belong to the organization.

Paperwork and procedures for employing staff

Prior to recruitment

The following points are important to consider.

- Do you have the appropriate authority to go ahead and fill the vacancy? It is unhelpful to offer a job only to find that it has been frozen by financial cutbacks.
- Draw up a *job description* prior to employing staff, it helps you to be clear about what is required and prevents doubts about the duties at a later date.

- Put the terms and conditions for the post in writing prior to employment. You can then be clear about the obligations and rights of the employee. It will help considerably to reduce any later disagreements. It is also legally required for most full-time employees within 13 weeks of the start of their employment.
- It is advisable to inform staff of your intentions ahead of actions being taken to recruit new staff. You should explain how the post fits in with existing responsibilities. Equally, explain if there are likely delays in the refilling of existing posts.

Advertising

If a new employee is to be introduced into existing staffing arrangements, it is essential that the method of selection is perceived to be reasonably fair. This generally means advertising the vacancy. Word of mouth has the advantage of being cheap and possibly speedy. It has the disadvantage of limiting the range of applicants from which to choose and leaving the manager open to accusations of either discrimination or nepotism.

Advertising may be local or national. Generally, senior positions are better advertised nationally, if possible. Local advertisements can be successfully used for more junior posts. Advertising in the *Physiotherapy Journal* or *Therapy Weekly* will generally achieve a range of applicants. Whether local or national, or even internal, advertising ensures that any existing staff who wish to make an application have the opportunity to do so. It prevents later conflicts.

Writing advertisements

It is cheaper to advertise than use an agency. Just look at the other advertisements in the journal or paper of your choice and use them as a model. Alternatively, use your personnel department, but check carefully what is put in advertisements. Make sure that you include the job title, a brief statement of the duties, if it is part-time and, probably, the salary on offer. It should also include the name and address of your hospital, an appropriate telephone number and a closing date for applications.

Discrimination in advertisements

In both the advertisement and the interview, there are some simple rules you *must* follow to stay on the right side of the law:

- do not discriminate on racial grounds;
- do not discriminate on the grounds of sex or marital status;

- pay equal salaries to men or women applicants;
- do not discriminate because of trade union or non-trade union membership.

Selection interviews

Selecting through a formal interview process is both a sensible approach and a legal protection against claims of unfair discrimination. It provides the opportunity for the manager and any other members of an interview panel to probe in depth into the applicant's suitability for a particular post. It is a two-way process where the applicant is trying to convince the organization to employ her and, at the same time, the organization is trying to sell itself as a suitable place for employment. It provides a good opportunity to be clear about the terms of the post on offer (to avoid later misunderstanding), along with any further explanation of the duties expected.

It helps if the following steps are taken:

- Ask for formal curricula vitae (CV) or application forms completed by applicants.
- Check out references. It may be sensible not just to check her own referees, but also to check up with previous employers. This can be done by letter, but may also be effectively done by sending a letter and following up with a telephone call.
- Remember the requirements for State Registration for physiotherapists who are employed in the NHS. The Regulations (NHS Professions Supplementary to Medicine 1974)[1] stipulate that no physiotherapist shall be employed unless that person is registered with the appropriate board. This restriction does not exist for physiotherapists employed outside of the NHS in private hospitals or businesses.

Legal requirements in making an offer

Once you have made up your mind whom to employ follow these guidelines.

- Write a formal offer letter, which may confirm a verbal offer.
- Put into the letter, or into the documents attached, all the terms and conditions of the post and a copy of the written job description.
- State the date on which you expect the new appointee to start, if this is known to you.
- Ask the new appointee to sign a second copy of the letter and return it to you with the confirmation that they have accepted the offer. This then forms the written basis of the Contract of Employment.
- It is essential that the offer letter, terms of employment, the CV, the job description, and any other relevant documents are filed away in a safe place. They may be needed later.

Contracts of Employment

Physiotherapy Managers act on behalf of their employers. A Contract of Employment is a written or a verbal legal agreement is entered into between the employer and the employee which defines the rights and duties of both. A Contract of Employment, like any other, is made up of three ingredients:

1 the offer of employment, through the advertisement and interview, ending in the offer of the post;
2 acceptance of employment;
3 payment or consideration; this is the remuneration for the skill and service given to the employer. It is the absence of payment which means that hospital volunteers do not have contracts of employment.

A contract can be an entirely verbal agreement. The fact that there is no written document does not mean that a contract does not exist. However, it is usual to put the contract into written form as often as possible. If it comes to a legal challenge later, the courts or Industrial Tribunals will prefer the written terms of a contract, unless there is clear evidence that something else has been subsequently agreed. It is, therefore, important to put the terms of the offer in writing and to keep a record. It has already been emphasized that after 13 weeks staff have a legal right to demand certain written terms.

The Contract of Employment is unlikely to be a single written document. It is broader than this and may well include:

- Written terms and conditions, including offer letters.
- What is said in the advertisment, for example, 'we guarantee that you will move to the next grade within one year'.
- Any specific additional terms agreed in the interview, such as that the employee could have every third Thursday off as unpaid leave to train as an Olympic swimmer.
- The terms of any Whitley agreements or PRB awards which apply to the particular post. Details of the agreements do not need to be given to the employee. They can be referred to in an available handbook of agreements.
- Any subsequent formal agreement reached in talks between you and the employee after employment, for instance that the physiotherapist can move to part-time instead of full-time working hours.

Any contract of employment has three principal terms which are:

1 *Expressed terms*: these are the arrangements talked about above in the interview or written documents including the salary, hours of work and so on.

2 *Implied terms*: these are things that are so obvious that it is usually not thought necessary to discuss them formally at the interview or to write them down. They include the employee's duties (*see* below) such as honesty and loyalty. But there may also be 'custom and practice', such as the wearing of uniform, which assumes that anyone joining that industry would know it as an implied term of his or her contract from the start.

3 *Imposed terms*: are specific terms imposed into a Contract of Employment by law and general legislation; for example, for a community physiotherapist to drive a car the law requires him or her to hold a driving licence. Equally, the Health & Safety at Work Act aims to ensure that both the employer and the employee undertake safe practices at work.

Employer's duties: the common law expects that the employer should:

- behave reasonably in employment matters;
- pay the agreed wages;
- take reasonable care of the employee's safety;
- practice good industrial relations by having clear disciplinary procedures and grievance procedures;
- comply with legal requirements on discrimination, pregnancy, dismissal and part-time staff.

Employee's duties: whatever the written statement in other documents, there are certain duties which employees have towards the employer under common law. Failure to adhere to these can result in disciplinary action. However, the circumstances of any alleged breach should be taken into account. Employees should:

- obey all reasonable and lawful orders;
- not be involved in misconduct;
- not disclose confidential information about the employer's business to others, but note that there are legal requirements concerning the disclosure about the abuse of patients in health care, professional requirements about appropriate conduct and the right of recognized representatives to undertake their duties;
- use reasonable skill and care in the work;
- take care of the employer's property;
- give faithful and honest service.

Legal rights to written terms and conditions

It has already been suggested that it is wise for employers to draw up written terms and conditions of employment prior to interviews taking place. However, the employer is legally obliged to give a written statement of the main terms and conditions of employment within 13 weeks of employment starting, for staff working more than 16 hours per week. Staff working between eight and 16 hours per week acquire this right after five years service.

After 13 weeks, you are legally obliged to provide information of the following terms and conditions; if you do not have such an arrangement or terms you simply say so in the statement.

- *Pay*: how it is worked out, monthly or weekly, and probably the salary grade to which it is linked.
- *Hours of work*: normal start and finishing times plus total hours per week.
- *Paid holidays*: (including Bank Holidays) and how this is calculated.
- *Sick pay entitlement*: (including Statutory Sick Pay).
- *Pension and pension schemes*: including a statement of whether you are contracted out of the State Pension Scheme. If you do not have a separate pension scheme for staff, you are by definition not contracted out. Most NHS staff are contracted out of the State scheme.
- *Period of notice*: the period of notice to be given on either side must be stated.
- *The job title*.
- *Information*: about any disciplinary rules and grievance procedures, including to whom the employee can appeal if she is dissatisfied with any disciplinary decision. In the NHS the GWC and Health Authority agreements provide this information.
- You may decide to provide additional information about uniform, clothing allowance or other benefits which are provided.
- Written terms would also give the opportunity to include any flexible terms that were thought appropriate.

Changes to contract terms

Contracts are legal, enforceable agreements, but they are rarely fixed and unchanging. Contracts may have built-in elements of flexibility; they can be varied by mutual agreement, by collective agreement, by the acceptance of a change in working practices or by the employer terminating the existing contracts. Various methods of changing contracts are explored below.

Change by individual agreement

This is the commonest form of contract change—by mutual agreement—between the employer and the employee. An employee who has worked for you for some time could request that the starting time should be changed from 9 to 10 a.m. each morning to enable her to drop her children off at school. If you agree to this change, this becomes a new contractual term.

Contractual right to vary

This right may be explicit or implied. A job description, for example, may make it clear that the list of duties included was not meant to be exhaustive and that the individual physiotherapist might be asked to undertake other appropriate duties. Equally, many Health Authorities write into their contracts a requirement for staff to be willing to move to other Units or hospitals within the Health Authority. This may give the right to move someone depending on whether or not such moves were ever expected of staff.

However, a recent High Court case (United Bank Ltd v. Akhtar 1989)[2] has made it very clear that the courts will imply a strong test of 'reasonable behaviour' by the employer into any such request to move. In this case, Mr Akhtar was required to move from one branch of his bank to another branch at the other end of the country, on a permanent basis, with only one week's notice; he was not given any removal expenses or other assistance and he faced taking care of a seriously ill wife. Although his contract appeared to give the employer the power to do this, the court deemed this to be completely unreasonable behaviour by the employer, who was obliged to pay compensation to Mr Akhtar.

Variation by union agreement

A new collective agreement, such as an NHS Whitley agreement, generally has the automatic effect of amending the Contract of Employment of the staff covered by it. The annual agreement on pay, for example, will normally automatically amend the Contract of Employment of staff employed by Health Authorities. Other terms and conditions can be similarly amended by collective agreements. The new SGTs in the NHS will have the right to engage in their own negotiations. Thus, although the national agreements may not apply, any local agreements may result in a variation of the Contract of Employment of the staff covered by it.

Acceptance of variations by the conduct of the employee

If a contractual term is changed by an employer and the employee continues to work under those conditions without protest, they will legally eventually be considered to have acquiesced to them. However, in another case (Rigby v. Ferodo Ltd 1987)[3] in the House of Lords, an employer (Ferodo) wished to reduce payments to Mr Rigby and other members of staff. The employee and his trade union refused the change of pay, and put this refusal in writing.

Ferodo paid less. Mr Rigby and his workmates stayed on and with the backing of their trade union sued the company for the reduction in salary. The House of Lords held that there was no agreed variation, either expressed or implied. Therefore Ferodo Ltd had breached the Contract of Employment and Mr Rigby was entitled to damages equivalent to the money he should originally have got.

Variation by termination of contract

This is a 'unilateralist' method of variation which is contrary to good industrial relations and can be extremely risky for the employer. It amounts to the employer giving notice—either by the appropriate time or money in lieu—to terminate the existing contract and then offering a new contract with the new term included in it. If the employees have the required length of service (two years in most cases), they will be able to go to an Industrial Tribunal and make a claim for unfair dismissal. Even if service is shorter, such action is likely to provoke serious conflict with the trade union representing the members. It is far more effective to achieve change by mutual agreement, unless contractual flexibility has been previously built into the basic contract.

Notice periods

The law requires the employer to provide a certain amount of notice to the employee in order to terminate the Contract of Employment.

The employer must give employees:

1 One week's notice if the employee has been with them for one month, but less than two years.
2 Two weeks' notice if the employee has been with them for two years.
3 An extra week's notice for each extra week the employee has been with them, up to a maximum of 12 weeks' notice.
4 If the employee's contract specifies a longer notice period, the longer period applies, for example, if three months' notice of termination is stated from the beginning of the contract, that will apply even if the employer decides to terminate the contract after only one week.

Failure to provide the appropriate notice or pay the appropriate amount in lieu of notice is known as wrongful dismissal and the employer can be sued for the money owing through the County Court (Court of Session in Scotland).

● The employee does not have to give the same amount of notice. By law, he/she is only required to give one week's notice if employed for more than a month. However, the employer may put into the terms of the original contract a requirement for one month's notice—the usual requirement—or more if this is considered necessary.

- It is possible to employ staff on Fixed Term Contracts of Employment. This would specify employment for a set period of six months, one year, two or three years. Such contracts now exist in the NHS, particularly for General Managers who are on three-year 'rolling' contracts; this means that at any given time they normally have another two years of their contract to run.

Fixed Term Contracts may be appropriate if the employer is certain that this is a short-term post for which longer term funding cannot be guaranteed, for example, a research project. The difficulty with using Fixed Term Contracts for other sorts of posts is that it promotes insecurity among staff and makes team-work difficult. There is a serious national shortage of physiotherapists to fill available vacancies, and 'temporary' staff are liable to leave at any time for a more secure post. If the employer decides to terminate the contract early, the employer may be liable to pay the individual for the remaining period of his Fixed Term Contract. This could amount, in some circumstances to two or more years' salary.

Grievance and dispute procedures

Grievance procedures are designed to deal with individual complaints. Disputes procedures are for collective complaints. Many Health Authorities and other employers have separate procedures for grievances and disputes. The Employment Protection (Consolidation) Act 1978 (referred to as the EPCA) requires notice to be given to employees of any existing procedures for dealing with complaints and the person to whom appeals should be made.

A grievance procedure is extremely useful in providing a formal mechanism to resolve problems which could either result in disputes and discontent among staff or to members of staff leaving employment unnecessarily. It also provides an opportunity for a management decision affecting the terms of employment of individuals to be reviewed by a more senior manager.

Grievance and disputes procedures are normally collectively negotiated at local level. In the NHS, Section 32 of the GWC agreements gives the right of appeal to individuals with a grievance about the application of a Whitley agreement, first to the DHA, if that fails on to the RHA and ultimately to the National Whitley Council. It is uncommon—with the exception of Clinical Nurses grading appeals—for appeals to progress beyond DHA level.

Managers should make themselves well acquainted with the grievance and the disputes procedure which operates in their authority or employing organization. However, the vast majority of individual grievances are settled by informal discussions between the employee and the manager concerned.

Disciplinary procedures and termination of employment

Adequate disciplinary procedures are an essential part of good employment practice. They are designed to protect both the employee and the employer against either arbitrary action or against charges of a failure to adhere to a reasonable procedure. This has been re-enforced by a recent court case (Polkey v. A. E. Dayton (Services) Ltd 1987)[4] which establishes that the failure to adhere to a fair procedure is likely to make a dismissal for any members of staff—who have the appropriate service to go to an Industrial Tribunal—automatically unfair. This case has reversed previous legal decisions which had limited the requirements of fairness. The Code of Practice published in 1977 by the Advisory Conciliation and Arbitration Service (ACAS)—and included in their 1987 ACAS handbooks (ACAS 1987)[5]—lists the essential features of disciplinary procedures. Most NHS disciplinary procedures, which have been negotiated by staff and employers locally, have the main features of the Code incorporated into them.

The procedures indicate a series of stages through which any action should be taken. This normally includes the opportunity for informal discussion, proper formal investigation, verbal warnings, two or more written warnings and, eventually, dismissal. An appeals process to the employing authority will also be built into the procedure.

Staff who are dismissed in accordance with the procedure may still have a right to go to an Industrial Tribunal to claim unfair dismissal. The current requirement is that an employee must have two years full-time employment with their current employer, or five years employment in the case of part-time staff working between eight and 16 hours per week.

However, if the employer dismisses somebody on the grounds of sex, marriage, race or trade union activities, he is are liable to be automatically guilty of unfair dismissal, no matter how short the service of the employer or employee concerned. The lesson is not to discriminate.

Future changes in NHS industrial relations

Physiotherapy Managers face the prospect of enormous change in industrial relations throughout the 1990s. Pressures towards decentralization of management in the NHS, tighter financial controls through competitive contracts, increasing shortages of staff in particular areas, and the likelihood that the Government will continue to take a major political interest in controlling the activities of health employers with all the major influences on the process of that change. It will inevitably mean that Physiotherapy Managers, along with others in the NHS, will be obliged to take an active interest in the conduct of industrial relations and methods of negotiations with staff in ways which have never been necessary in the past.

In the forefront of this change will be the SGTs. It is likely that the first 50 of these semi-independent NHS Trusts will officially come into existence on the 1 April 1991. They may well be followed by a 'second wave' in 1992. Whether or not any further Trusts are created will depend crucially on the outcome of the next general election. If the Conservatives succeed in being re-elected, the process of change towards large numbers of SGTs will accelerate.

The Trusts have been given the right under the 1990 NHS Act to negotiate or determine their own terms and conditons of employment for staff, separate to those laid down in the national agreements or PRB recommendations. Existing staff who are transferred into the Trust on 1 April 1990 will continue to have their *existing* Whitley terms and conditions protected under clause 6 of the Act. However that protection only applies to existing staff and existing agreements on the transfer date of 31 March 1990. Therefore, it probably does not include new agreements (such as the 1991 Review Body Award) unless the Trusts separately agree to apply them. These transfer terms do not apply to new staff employed by the SGTs after 1 April 1991. Such staff could be offered new employment packages which are less favourable or more favourable than the existing Whitley conditions. This could be an immediate source of conflict in physiotherapy departments or create difficulty in recruiting already scarce physiotherapy staff. It could set one staff member against another. It could also be a major source of conflict with the trade unions if it becomes a method of undermining existing national standards. The majority of Trusts on the first wave have indicated that they will apply existing conditions for new staff until such time as they establish new agreements or employment packages. Nevertheless, there may be a number of hospitals that will not operate in this way.

Local bargaining is likely to become an increasingly common reality as the decade progresses. There is considerable pressure from the NHS Management Executive on the Trusts to engage in local bargaining as soon as possible. Initially only a few of the Trusts will have the managerial IR skills or experience or the desire to take up local bargaining. However, within a few years, this initial hesitancy will disappear to be replaced by full blown local bargaining on the private sector model. This could involve physiotherapy and other NHS managers in an enormous cultural and organizational change which could potentially increase conflict with staff if it is not properly manged. Issues such as the right of any or all of the existing 30 Whitley staff organizations to be 'recognized' for local pay bargaining are likely to appear at an early stage in the light of the SGTs. A large amount of additional time and effort will be taken up with such local bargaining.

The current national problems about the restrictions of Government limits on pay could increasingly be replaced by local conflicts over new cash limits dictated by the local contract prices for work negotiated between NHS Trusts and the NHS DHA 'providers'. It may be argued that national pay bargaining in the NHS helps to defuse conflict. Local bargaining will lead at some point to industrial action by large or small groups of staff in order to put on pressure for a better deal. Managers will have to learn to cope with this.

The increasing emphasis in SGT pay packages will be upon 'individual' employment packages built to meet local need and local shortages of staff. Work flexibility, PRP; the elimination of additional pay allowances, skill mix and job substitution will all become issues on which managers will have to negotiate.

In turn such pressures are likely to lead to SGTs forming employers' federations, and trade unions increasingly developing closer methods of working together and exchanging information. In the view of some, the future will involve fewer NHS staff who will be more highly paid and work harder. This assumes that staff are not working hard now!

One dream is unlikely to become a reality, SGTs – short of complete privatization – will not become free of Government influence and Government control. The Treasury and the politicians have far too much at stake to give local Trusts complete freedom to operate the business as they see fit, particularly in the area of wages and potential industrial conflicts. The future will not be easy for Physiotherapy Managers but it will certainly be interesting.

References

Chapter 1

1. Handy, C. (1986) *Understanding Organizations*. Penguin Business Library, Middx.
2. Barnard, C. (1938) The Functions of the Executive. In: Koontz, H., O'Donnell, C. and Weirich, M. *Management*. McGraw Hill, Japan, 1984.
3. Armstrong, M. (1986) *A Handbook of Management Techniques*. Kogan Page, London, p. 15.
4. Drucker, P. (1968) *The Practice of Management*. Pan Books, London.
5. Drucker, P. (1968) *The Practice of Management*. Pan Books, London.
6. Jones, R. J. (1989) *Physiotherapy and its Management in the National Health Service Districts of England and Wales*. MPhil Thesis, p. 165.
7. Jones, R. J. (1989) *Physiotherapy and its Management in the National Health Service Districts of England and Wales*. MPhil Thesis, p. 167.
8. Jones, R. J. (1989) *Physiotherapy and its Management in the National Health Service Districts of England and Wales*. MPhil Thesis, p. 179.
9. Williams, J. (1986) *Monitoring Effectiveness in Physiotherapy Services*. Report of two participative workshops—No. 2, Doncaster Health Authority.
10. Brooks, R. (Editor) (1986) *Management Budgeting in the NHS*. Health Services Manpower Review, Keele.
11. Williams, J. (1986) *Measuring Efficiency in Physiotherapy Services*. Report of two participative workshops—No. 3, Doncaster Health Authority.
12. Williams, J. (1986) *Measuring Efficiency in Physiotherapy Services*. Report of two participative workshops—No. 3, Doncaster Health Authority.

Chapter 2

1. Friedson, E. (1970) *Profession of Medicine*. Dodd Mead & Co, New York.
2. Carr-Saunders, A. M. & Wilson, P. A. (1933) *The Professions*. The Clarendon Press, Oxford.
3. Greenwood, E. (1957) Attributes of a Profession. *Social Work*, 2, 45–55.
4. Wilensky, H. L. (1964) The Professionalization of Everyone. *American Journal of Sociology*, 70(2), 137–158.

5. Johnson, T. J. (1972) *Professions and Power.* MacMillan Press, London.
6. Wickstead, J. H. (1948) *The Growth of a Profession.* Edward Arnold & Co, London.
7. Mercer, J. (1978) Physiotherapy as a Profession. *Physiotherapy,* 66(6), 80–184.
8. Goode, W. J. (1969) The Theoretical Limits of Professionalization. In Etzioni, A. (Editor), *The Semi Professions and their Organization.* The Free Press, New York.
9. Etzioni, A. (1979) *The Semi Professions and their Organization: Teachers, Nurses, Social Workers.* Collier MacMillan, London.
10. Friedson, E. (1971) *Professional Dominance.* Atherton Press.

Chapter 3

1. Ministry of Health RHB(49)114, HMC(49)93. (1949) Memorandum sent by Ministry of Health to Regional Health Boards, Hospital Management Committees and Board of Governors of Teaching Hospitals.
2. DHSS (1951) *Reports of the Committees on Medical Auxiliaries—The Cope Report*—Cmd. 8188. HMSO, London.
3. DHSS (1951) *Reports of the Committees on Medical Auxiliaries—The Cope Report*—Cmd. 8188. HMSO, London.
4. Larkin, G. (1983) *Occupational Monopoly and Modern Medicine,* Tavistock Publications, London.
5. DHSS (1951) *Reports of the Committees on Medical Auxiliaries—The Cope Report*—Cmd. 8188. HMSO, London.
6. DHSS (1951) *Reports of the Committees on Medical Auxiliaries—The Cope Report*—Cmd. 8188. HMSO, London.
7. DHSS (1972) *Rehabilitation: Report of a Sub-Committee of the Standing Medical Advisory Committee—Tunbridge Report.* HMSO, London.
8. DHSS (1972) *Rehabilitation: Report of a Sub-Committee of the Standing Medical Advisory Committee—Tunbridge Report.* HMSO, London.
9. DHSS (1972) *Rehabilitation: Report of a Sub-Committee of the Standing Medical Advisory Committee—Tunbridge Report* HMSO, London.
10. DHSS (1972) Statement by the Committee on the Remedial Professions. HMSO, London.
11. Patrick, M. (1986) Physiotherapy—My Chosen Career. *Journal of the Association of District and Superintendent Chartered Physiotherapists,* 6, 6–10.

12. DHSS (1973) *The Remedial Professions*. A report by a Working Party set up in March 1973 by the Secretary of State for Social Services—The McMillan Report. HMSO, London.
13. DHSS (1973) *The Remedial Professions*. A report by a Working Party set up in March 1973 by the Secretary of State for Social Services—The McMillan Report. HMSO, London.
14. DHSS (1973) *The Remedial Professions*. A report by a Working Party set up in March 1973 by the Secretary of State for Social Services—The McMillan Report. HMSO, London.
15. DHSS (1973) *The Remedial Professions*. A report by a Working Party set up in March 1973 by the Secretary of State for Social Services—The McMillan Report. HMSO, London.
16. DHSS (1973) *The Remedial Professions*. A report by a Working Party set up in March 1973 by the Secretary of State for Social Services—The McMillan Report. HMSO, London.
17. DHSS (1972) *Management Arrangements for the Re-organised National Health Service—The Grey Book*. HMSO, London.
18. DHSS (1972) *Management Arrangements for the Re-organised National Health Service—The Grey Book*. HMSO, London.
19. DHSS (1972) *Management Arrangements for the Re-organised National Health Service—The Grey Book*. HMSO, London.
20. DHSS (1972) *Management Arrangements for the Re-organised National Health Service—The Grey Book*. HMSO, London.
21. DHSS (1974) *The Remedial Professions and Linked Therapies*. HSC(IS)101.
22. DHSS (1974) *The Remedial Professions and Linked Therapies*. HSC(IS)101.
23. DHSS (1975) *Report of the Committee of Inquiry into the Pay and Related Conditions of Service of the Professions Supplementary to Medicine and Speech Therapists—Halsbury Report*. HMSO, London.
24. DHSS (1975) Advance Letter (PTA) 20/75.
25. DHSS (1975) DS 331/75. *Designation of Therapists*.
26. DHSS (1977) *Report of the Sub-group on the Organization of the Remedial Professions in the National Health Service*. HMSO, London.
27. DHSS (1979) *Health Services Development, Management of the Remedial Professions in the NHS*. HC(79)19.
28. DHSS (1978) Draft Health Circular on Management of the Remedial Professions in the NHS. Notes by DHSS.
29. Jones, R. J. (1987) The Development of Physiotherapy Management in the NHS. In *The CSP Source Book*. Parke Sutton, Norwich, pp. 48–52.
30. DHSS (1977) *Health Services Development—Relationship between the Medical and Remedial Professions*. HC(77)33.

31. DHSS (1977) *Health Services Development—Relationship between the Medical and Remedial Professions*. HC(77)33.
32. The Royal Commission on the National Health Service 1979—*Merrison Report*—Cmd. 7615, HMSO, London.
33. DHSS (1979) *Patients First*. HMSO, London.
34. DHSS (1980) *Health Services Development, Structure and Management*. HC(80)8.
35. DHSS (1980) *Health Services Development, Structure and Management*. HC(80)8.
36. CSP (1986) *Rules of Professional Conduct*. CSP, London.
37. Flew, A. (Editor) (1984) *A Dictionary of Philosophy*. Pan Reference, London.
38. DHSS (1989) *Working for Patients*—the White Paper. HMSO, London.
39. CSP (1989) *Note of meeting with David Mellor, Minister of State for Health*.
40. CSP (1989) *Note of meeting with David Mellor, Minister of State for Health*.

Chapter 4

1. DHSS/Griffiths (1983) *National Health Service Management Inquiry—Griffiths Report*. HMSO, London.
2. DHSS (1984) *Health Services Management—Implementation of the NHS Management Inquiry*. HC(84)13.
3. Hansard (1983) *Written Answers in Hansard*, 3.2., p. 181.
4. DHSS/Griffiths (1983) *National Health Service Management Inquiry—Griffiths Report*. HMSO, London.
5. DHSS (1972) *Management Arrangements for the Reorganized National Health Service—the Grey Book*. HMSO, London.
6. DHSS (1972) *Rehabilitation: Report of a Sub-Committee of the Standing Medical Advisory Committee—the Tunbridge Report*. HMSO, London.
7. DHSS/Griffiths (1983) *National Health Service Management Inquiry—Griffiths Report*. HMSO, London.
8. DHSS/Griffiths (1983) *National Health Service Management Inquiry—Griffiths Report*. HMSO, London.
9. Evans, T. & Maxwell, R. (1984) *Griffiths: Challenge and Response*—Evidence to Select Committee on Social Services, Kings Fund, London, p. 3.
10. DHSS/Griffiths (1983) *National Health Service Management Inquiry—Griffiths Report*. HMSO, London.

11. The Royal Commission on the National Health Service (1979) *Merrison Report*—Cmd. 7615. HMSO, London.
12. DHSS/Griffiths (1983) *National Health Service Management Inquiry —Griffiths Report*. HMSO, London.
13. French, D. & Saward, H. (1984) *A Dictionary of Management*. Pan Reference, London.
14. DHSS (1975) *Designation of Therapists*. DS331/75.
15. Dixon, M. (1983) The Organisation and Structure of Units. In I. Wickings (Editor) *Effective Unit Management*. Kings Fund, London.

Chapter 5

1. Department of Health (1989) *Working for Patients*. Cmd. 555, HMSO, London.
2. Department of Health (1989) *Caring for People. Community Care in the Next Decade and Beyond*. Cmd. 849, HMSO, London.
3. DHSS (1987) *Promoting Better Health*. Cmd. 249, HMSO, London.
4. DHSS (1988) *Community Care: Agenda for Action*. HMSO, London.
5. DHSS (1988) *Community Care: Agenda for Action*. HMSO, London.

Chapter 7

1. Körner E. (1985) *A Further Report on the Collection and Use of Information about the Community in the NHS* (4th Report). DHSS Steering Group on Health Service Information, HMSO, London.
2. CSP/COT/DHSS (1986) *Clinical and Managerial Information Systems for Physiotherapy and Occupational Therapy Report (Yellow Book)*. CSP Professional Affairs Department.
3. Department of Health Information Management Group (April 1990) *Recommendations of the Working Group on Indicators for the Community Health Service*, p. 2.
4. Department of Health Information Management Group (April 1990) *Recommendations of the Working Group on Indicators for the Community Health Service*, p. 30.
5. DHSS (1986) *Resource Management (Management Budgeting) for Health Authorities*. HN(86)34.
6. Department of Health—NHS Management Executive (February 1990) *Resource Management*.
7. IBM (1990) *Resource Management*, p. 1.
8. Williams J. I. (1987) Resource Management. *Physiotherapy Journal* 73(10), 531–532.

9. Department of Health (1989) Technical Guidance Notes 'Casemix Management'. February 1989. In *Information Package—Acute Hospitals*. Technical Guidance Notes for Roll-Out Sites, p. 21.
10. Department of Health (1989) Technical Guidance Notes 'Casemix Management'. February 1989. In *Information Package—Acute Hospitals*. Technical Guidance Notes for Roll-Out Sites, p. 23.
11. Read, J. D & Benson, T. J. R. (1986) Comprehensive Coding. *British Journal of Healthcare Computing*, 3(2) 22–25.
12. Department of Health (1990) *Framework for Information Systems: The Next Steps*. Pre-publication Draft, p. 56.
13. Department of Health (1989) Diagnosis Related Groups TGN3. In *Resource Management Initiative Information Package—Acute Hospitals*. Technical Guidance Notes for Roll-Out Sites, p. 15.
14. DHSS (1986) *Resource Management Management Budgeting for Health Authorities*.
15. Department of Health Information Management Group (June 1990) *Working for Patients 'Information Systems: The Next Steps'*, p. 3.
16. Department of Health (June 1990) *Framework for Information Systems: The Next Steps*.
17. Department of Health (1990) *Framework for Information Systems: The Next Steps*, p. 33.
18. Department of Health (1990) *Framework for Information Systems: The Next Steps*, p. 33.
19. Williams, J. I. (1990) *Resource Management Workshop Papers*.
20. Chartered Society of Physiotherapy (1990) Principles on Information Systems and Resource Management. *Physiotherapy Journal*, 76(2), 74.

Chapter 9

1. Maxwell, R. J. (1984) Quality assessment in health. *British Medical Journal*, 288(1), 470–471.
2. *Physiotherapy Services: A Basis for Development of Standards*. King's Fund Centre, London, 1987.
3. Shaw, C. (1984) *Medical Audit—A Hospital Handbook*. King's Fund Centre, London.

Chapter 11

1. DHSS (1986) *Individual Performance Review*. PM(86)10.
2. DHSS (1986) *General Managers—Arrangements for the Introduction of Performance-Related Pay* PM(86)11.

Chapter 12

1. Handy, C. (1981) *Understanding Organisations*. Penguin Business Library, Middx.
2. Handy, C. (1981) *Understanding Organisations*. Penguin Business Library, Middx.
3. South East Thames Regional Health Authority (1989) Working Groups.
4. Trent RHA Manpower Planning—Physiotherapy (1989) An examination of supply and demand issues.
5. Loomis, J. (1985) Evaluating Clinical Competence of Physical Therapy Students Part 1 & 2 The Development of an Instrument. *Physiotherapy*, Canada, March/April.
6. Carey, D. (1983) Competence—Can it be Assessed? *Physiotherapy Journal*, September.
7. Ford, S. G. (1985) Clinical Competence of Physiotherapy Students: Development of an Assessment Form. *NZ Journal of Physiotherapy*, December.
8. Levine, H. G. (1985) *Medicine. A Model Paediatric Clerkship in Evaluating Clinical Competence in the Health Professions*. Morgan, M. and Irby, D. (Editors) St. Louis C V, Mosby.
9. Littlefield, J. H., Harrington, J. T., Anthracite, N. E. & German, R. E. (1981) A description and four-year Analysis of a Clinical Clerkship Evaluation System. *Journal of Medical Education*, 53, 55–58.
10. Department of Health (1989) *Working for Patients*—The White Paper.

Chapter 13

1. Atkinson, H. W. (1988) Head in the Clouds, Feet on the Ground. *Physiotherapy*, 74(11), 542–547.
2. Greenwood, E. (1957) Attributes of a Profession. In H. M. Vollmer and D. L. Mills (Editors) *Professionalization*. Prentice Hall.
3. Brook, N. & Parry, A. W. (1985) The Influence of Higher Education on the Assessment of Students of Physiotherapy. *Assessment and Evaluation in Higher Education*, 10(2) 131–146.
4. Partridge, C. & Barnitt, R. (1986) *Research Guidelines: A Handbook for Therapists*. Heinemann Physiotherapy.
5. Shulman, L. (1981) Disciplines of Inquiry in Education: an Overview. *Educational Researcher*, 10(6), 5–12.
6. Patton, M. Q. (1980) *Qualitative Evaluation Methods*. Sage Publications.

7. Reid, N. G. & Boore, J. R. P. (1987) *Research Methods and Statistics in Health Care*. Edward Arnold.
8. Partridge, C. & Barnitt, R. (1986) *Research Guidelines: A Handbook for Therapists*. Heinemann, Oxford.
9. The Chartered Society of Physiotherapy (1990) *Guideline 10: Literature Search: What to Look For and Where to Go*.
10. Partridge, C. & Barnitt, R. (1986) *Research Guidelines: A Handbook for Therapists*. Heinemann, Oxford.
11. Cobb, A. K. and Hagemaster, J. N. (1987) Ten Criteria for Evaluating Qualitative Research Proposals. *Journal of Nursing Education*, 26, 4.
12. The Chartered Society of Physiotherapy (1990) *Guideline 11: Sources of Funding and How to Apply*.

Chapter 14

1. McCarthy, W. (1976) *Making Whitley Work*. HMSO, London, p. 11.
2. Clegg, H. A. & Chester, T. E. (1957) *Wages Policy and the Health Service*. Basil Blackwell, Oxford.
3. National Health Service Act 1977, amended by Schedule 6 of the National Health Service Act, 1983.
4. Pay Review Body (1987) *Review Body for Nursing Staff, Midwives, Health Visitors, and Professions Allied to Medicine*. Fourth Report on Professions Allied to Medicine, HMSO, London.

Chapter 15

1. NHS (Professions Supplementary to Medicine) Regulations (1974) SI, 1974, No. 496.
2. United Bank Ltd v. Akhtar (1989) Industrial Relations Law Reports 507.
3. Rigby v. Ferodo Ltd (1987) Industrial Relations Law Reports 517.
4. Polkey v. A. E. Dayton (Services) Ltd (1987) IRLR 503.
5. ACAS (1987) 'Discipline at Work—The ACAS Advisory Handbook'. Advisory Conciliation and Arbitration Service.

Index

accountability 9–10, 24, 53
ad hoc reports 75, 76–80
administrative staff 120–1
Advance Letters 165
advertisements, job 178–9
age, discrimination on grounds of 171
Agenda for Action 44, 46
aims and objectives 7
ancillary staff 120–1
audit, and quality assurance 109–11
autonomy 18–32

blanket referrals 56
budget statements 91

capital charges 47
care profiles 85
Caring for People 44
case management 46–7
case-mix management systems 85–6
case notes, as legal documents 55
Chartered Society of Massage and Medical
    Gymnastics 13–14
Chartered Society of Physiotherapy
    (CSP) 14–15
    and maintenance of ethical
        standards 29–30
    as a trade union 159–60
clerical staff 120–1
clinical autonomy 27–8
clinical diagnosis 30–1
clinical placements 133–4
    finance for 136–7
    policies on 136
Clinical Supervisor
    criteria for 134
    role 130–2
CMMS 85–6
coding systems 86–8
commissioning authorities 45–7
Committee on the Remedial
    Professions 20
    Statement by 21
compensation 53
competence 53
    assessment of 134–5
computer terminology, glossary 95–101
consensus management 33
consent 56–7

consumer satisfaction surveys 109
contracts 47–8
contracts of employment 180–2
    changes to terms 182–4
    fixed term 185
    termination of 184
Cope Report 18–19
cost, definition 90
costing exercises 93–4
costing of services 89–90
Council for Professions Supplementary to
    Medicine 15–16
criminal offences, and employment
    discrimination 172–3
criteria audit 111
CSP *see* Chartered Society of Physiotherapy

DHAs *see* District Health Authorities
diagnosis related groups 88
directly managed units 47
disciplinary procedures 186
discrimination in employment 170–3,
    178–9
dispute procedures 185–6
District Health Authorities (DHAs)
    as commissioning authorities 45
    responsibilities 52
District Physiotherapist 40–1, 42
    duties and responsibilities 2–6
    and general management 41, 43
    genesis of post 21–31
    impact of employment law on 169–74
    and research 139
DRGs 88
duty of care 52

Education Act 1981, physiotherapists'
    responsibilities under 58
education and training 14, 15
    finance 136–7
    in-service 115–16
    policies 136
    see also students
effectiveness 7–9
efficiency 7–9
employees 176
    duties 181
employers 177
    duties 181
employment law 169–74